# Demodex and Rosacea

# Demodex and Rosacea

Hui-Peng Huang
Director of Huang Hui-Peng Dermatology Clinic in Tainan, Taiwan

World Scientific
NEW JERSEY • LONDON • SINGAPORE • BEIJING • SHANGHAI • HONG KONG • TAIPEI • CHENNAI • TOKYO

*Published by*

World Scientific Publishing Co. Pte. Ltd.
5 Toh Tuck Link, Singapore 596224
*USA office:* 27 Warren Street, Suite 401-402, Hackensack, NJ 07601
*UK office:* 57 Shelton Street, Covent Garden, London WC2H 9HE

**British Library Cataloguing-in-Publication Data**
A catalogue record for this book is available from the British Library.

**DEMODEX AND ROSACEA**



ISBN 978-981-98-2788-6 (hardcover)
ISBN 978-981-98-2789-3 (ebook for institutions)
ISBN 978-981-98-2790-9 (ebook for individuals)

For any available supplementary material, please visit
https://www.worldscientific.com/worldscibooks/10.1142/14722#t=suppl

Typeset by Stallion Press
Email: enquiries@stallionpress.com

# Foreword 1

Recently, I received a request from Dr. Huang Hui-Peng, asking me to write a foreword for his new book, *Demodex* and Rosacea. When the Department of Dermatology of National Cheng Kung University Hospital was established in 1988, I was appointed the first chief physician of the department, and Dr. Huang was one of the first resident physicians. Dr. Huang performed excellently during his residency. After completing his training, I invited him to stay as an attending physician. However, because of family reasons, he decided to start his own business. That was about 30 years ago. Over the past years in my outpatient department (OPD) clinics at National Cheng Kung University Hospital, through the diagnostic results and treatments in Dr. Huang's referral notes, I was always gratified by his dedication to patients in the primary clinic and commitment toward healthcare quality.

In the past one or two decades, some dermatology clinics have hired nondermatologists to cover clinical shifts. To maintain healthcare quality, Dr. Huang has always managed the clinic shifts independently. What impressed me even more was that, as Dr. Huang mentioned in his preface, he became interested in association between *Demodex* and facial skin diseases, particularly rosacea in 2012. Later, he made in-depth observations and obtained insights into rosacea and other facial skin lesions. After years of hard work and joint clinical and pathological research with the Department of Dermatology of National Cheng Kung University Hospital, his achievements were published one after another during 2019–2022, and a total of six papers were published, including clinical diagnosis and differential diagnosis of rosacea. Two relatively simple methods to examine *Demodex* mite density (DMD) were developed (superficial needle-scraping method in 2019 and thumbnail-squeezing method in 2020), which can effectively evaluate and compare the DMD of rosacea and other facial skin lesions and then explore the association between *Demodex* overgrowth and rosacea (2021).

Subsequently, based on clinical experience, another three papers were published, providing detailed accounts of the effects of ivermectin and hydroxocobalamin on rosacea as well as the comparison of efficacy and side effects between different treatments.

Through Dr. Huang's detailed descriptions based on his years of research in this book, we can realize Dr. Huang's persistence on healthcare quality in the primary practice and his enthusiasm for clinical research. Among the dermatologists I know in the primary clinic, Dr. Huang is an excellent and extraordinary figure and an admirable clinical physician and medical researcher. His achievements make me, one of his teachers, and the Department of Dermatology of National Cheng Kung University Hospital proud. Thus, when Dr. Huang asked me to write a foreword for his new book, I felt honored and duty-bound.

His new book focuses on clinical and differential diagnosis of rosacea evaluation and comparison of DMD between rosacea and other facial skin lesions using a self-developed method to examine DMD, association between DMD and rosacea, and the effects of different treatments on rosacea. The detailed statements included in this book make it a valuable reference for physicians and patients. Because I have decided to write a foreword for his new book, I will not go into detail about its chapters. Here, I would like to provide a brief introduction to the clinical and pathological research on rosacea and demodicosis that we did at National Cheng Kung University Hospital before Dr. Huang started his research as a background to his work.

I came back from the US to National Cheng Kung University in 1988 at the invitation of the then Dean of National Cheng Kung University Medical School, Huang Kun-Yan, who was the in-charge of clinical services and research in the Department of Dermatology. Many years ago, when I was a resident physician at National Taiwan University, rosacea cases were still rare, and I had never diagnosed *Demodex* cases. After I joined National Cheng Kung University Hospital, through clinical and pathological observations, I gradually learned about the symptoms of these diseases and their diagnosis and treatments. In those days, the dermatology community in Taiwan knew little about or paid little attention to such diseases.

Rarely did these diseases appear in academic literature. Between 2004 and 2017, we successively compiled detailed data on clinical cases of rosacea and demodicosis and published eight articles on the clinical symptoms, diagnosis, treatments, and treatment of ineradicable and persistent facial erythema and erythema related to rosacea, as well as research reports on the clinical pathology of demodicosis. Based on clinical observations and treatment experience, we have become capable of discussing in depth on rosacea and demodicosis with Dr. Huang in recent years. I initiated the clinical research on rosacea and demodicosis in Taiwan, and these are the results of my work: the campaign to formally rename the Chinese disease name of rosacea in Taiwan from "wine dregs nose" to "rose spot" in 2004; two articles in 2005 emphasizing that rosacea is a facial disease commonly misdiagnosed; the diagnosis, treatment, and pathophysiology of rosacea; and the efficacy of oral carvedilol and topical brimonidine on rosacea. However, Dr. Huang's accumulation of experience and prowess through research on rosacea and *Demodex* has undoubtedly outpaced me. In my opinion, Dr. Huang is one of the leading experts in rosacea and *Demodex* both in Taiwan and in the international community and a pride of the dermatology community in Taiwan.

Looking back on the early years when I saw patients with rosacea in the OPD clinic, I often spent about 20 minutes on each patient. In addition to collecting information about their conditions, symptoms, predisposing factors, past medication treatments, and their response or efficacy, I also had to rule out any disease on their face prior to rosacea and associated complications. Thus, I could finally come up with the most appropriate diagnosis and treatment for rosacea and other diseases or complications. Some patients would develop persistent facial erythema, which was very difficult to treat. In addition to appearance problems, these patients would also feel hot and burning sensation in their faces, which resulted in severe mental and physical discomfort. I recall in the early days that some calls from the Chinese mainland reached my clinic for help after I published my successful experience in treating patients with ineradicable and persistent facial erythema. Fortunately, with the publication of our research findings, the dermatology community in Taiwan has significantly increased its attention to rosacea and its ability and experience in diagnosis and treatment of rosacea.

Therefore, in the last 10 years, many dermatologists across the country, including Lin Jeng-Hsien, another outstanding physician trained in the Department of Dermatology of National Cheng Kung University Hospital, have also devoted themselves to improving the diagnosis of rosacea and the quality of patient treatment. The achievement is fairly gratifying.

Modern medicine progresses rapidly and changes with each passing day. In addition to the many academic institutions and medical centers that are the main driving force in promoting research, there are physicians in the primary clinic, like Dr. Huang, who directly conduct in-depth clinical observations, are willing to work closely with medical centers, and continue to work hard to publish their research findings of many years. Their efforts to compile these articles into a book is even more precious, which enables more physicians and patients to find answers to their questions regarding these diseases. As such, I sincerely recommend this book and hope that more enthusiastic physicians in primary clinic will devote themselves to topics or fields that they have great interest and expertise in to conduct in-depth clinical research to benefit patients even further.

Professor of the Department of Dermatology,
National Cheng Kung University Medical School
Lee Yu-Yun

李玉雲

# Foreword 2

When I was a resident doctor, I thought that rosacea was a common skin disease among Westerners. Occasionally, when I saw patients with this disease, I treated them with oral tetracyclines and topical metronidazole. I also provided them with health education, such as using sunscreen and moisturizer and avoiding all worsening factors. As the number of patients increased in the waiting area of the clinic, we often saw patients with their faces fully covered in redness, to the extent that blood seemed to ooze out of their faces. These patients would keep fanning themselves or using hand-held electric fans. We often suspected that such patients had steroid-induced rosacea-like dermatosis. The patients were so helpless that they even developed neuroticism. Young resident physicians like us and attending physicians had no idea how to treat these patients, so we referred them to Prof. Lee Yu-Yun's OPD clinic, where patient meetings and health education speeches were conducted. To share clinical experience and treatment outcomes, Prof. Lee and Dr. Chia-Chi Hsu published their findings on application of carvedilol to treat persistent erythema and flushing of rosacea.

Dr. Huang Hui-Peng is 2 years senior to me in the university and currently works in the primary clinic. He is a dedicated physician who often spares time from his very tight clinical schedule to participate in the clinicopathological meetings on Wednesday afternoons. One day, Dr. Huang proposed to the chief resident to give him some time to share his research at the department's clinicopathological meeting. At that meeting, I realized how thorough Dr. Huang's research on *Demodex* was, with exquisite photos and videos recording the lifecycle of *Demodex*.

In the past decade, Dr. Huang has developed two innovative methods to examine *Demodex* and has made efforts to share them with colleagues in the Department of Dermatology. Moreover, the Department of Dermatology of National Cheng Kung University Hospital currently adopts his methods to examine *Demodex*, which proved to be satisfactory in the assessment of the *Demodex* count. After a series of studies and observations, combined with the understanding of the mechanisms of *Demodex* and their etiology and pathology, and together with the advent of new drugs, Dr. Huang can now provide the most appropriate treatment for patients with rosacea.

He also unsparingly shared his knowledge through lectures, seminars, health education activities, and social media to improve dermatologists' and patients' understanding of rosacea.

Doctors usually have limited time in their clinics for patients; thus, they cannot provide detailed explanations and instructions to patients and their family members. Therefore, Dr. Huang Hui-Peng compiled his rich clinical experience and published this book on rosacea in Taiwan, and this book covers the information he has accumulated over the past decade, including clinical experience, statistical data, published medical papers, and stories of patients with rosacea. I believe this book can facilitate a better understanding among dermatologists and patients with rosacea on the diagnosis, treatments, and health education of rosacea.

President of Taiwanese Dermatological Association
Associate Professor and Doctor, Department of Dermatology,
National Cheng Kung University Medical School
Chao Sheau-Chiou
趙曉秋

# Foreword 3

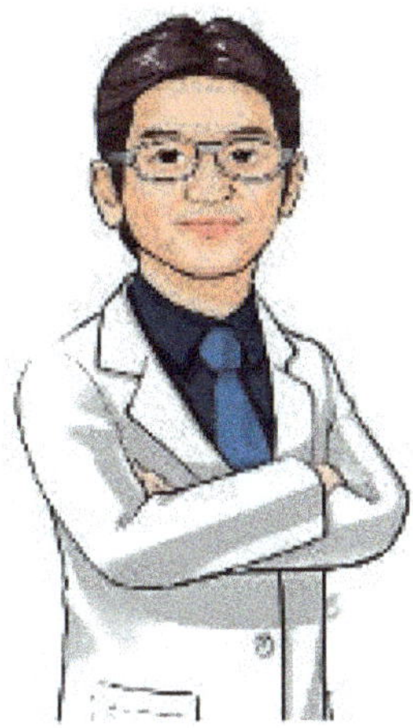

Rosacea is a common skin disease but is challenging to treat. It has been around since ancient times. It appears to be more prevalent among Caucasian Westerners, with symptoms such as red face and red nose. In severe cases, some patients may be mistaken for drinking alcohol. The symptoms of rosacea are sometimes very similar to eczema, allergies, and acne. It can easily relapse. In the past, we knew very little about the cause of this disease, had limited medications to treat it, and found it difficult to eradicate. With the advancement of medicine in recent years, many new medications have been developed. Topical drugs specific to flushing, erythema, anti-inflammation, and anti-*Demodex* have substantially improved the quality of life of patients with rosacea. However, good medicines depend on good diagnosis. To understand the causes for the exacerbation of different rosacea and determine whether excessive *Demodex* causes dermatitis, the doctors must have high professional clinical experience.

Dr. Huang has painstakingly studied rosacea for 10 years. He has conducted in-depth research on how *Demodex* causes skin inflammation, how to identify and diagnose it accurately, and how to provide more effective treatment. I admire his persistence in researching rosacea. In addition to treating patients, he could also spare time and effort to study this intractable skin disease. After accumulating abundant clinical treatment experience, he is willing to unsparingly share his knowledge with juniors by compiling his precious clinical experience into this book, which benefits numerous patients with rosacea.

Former Chief Physician at the Department of Dermatology
of Chang Gung Memorial Hospital
Chief Physician at the Department of
Dermatology and Immunology,
Taipei Chang Gung Memorial Hospital
Professor at College of Medicine of Chang Gung University
Chung Wen-Hung

# Foreword 4

March 25, 2018, is an important day.

It was the day when I was fortunate enough to attend the first class on how to examine *Demodex*, conducted by Dr. Huang Hui-Peng at his clinic. It was also the day I had a new understanding on how to treat rosacea. Before that, I had seen quite a few patients with rosacea in my clinic, and the treatment outcomes were fairly good. However, there were always some cases that showed unsatisfying outcomes or some with satisfying progress but a relapse before long.

Through this class, I realized that *Demodex* contributes substantially to the occurrence of rosacea; in addition, I was also amazed to know that Dr. Huang has been studying the association between rosacea and *Demodex* for many years. The concepts proposed by him are pioneering in Taiwan and still rarely discussed in international journals. Therefore, patients face difficulty comprehending the necessity of testing and treatment for *Demodex*, and dermatologists themselves exhibit a degree of skepticism toward this practice. It is conceivable that Dr. Huang must feel lonely and helpless in his research course.

However, pioneers are always solo fighters. After Dr. Huang compiled his findings into several research papers and made them available in international journals alongside dozens of academic seminars and speeches, more doctors in Taiwan accepted these concepts. Moreover, treatments based on these concepts have made satisfactory treatment outcomes accessible to many patients with chronic or recurrent rosacea, and such approaches have broadened the diagnostic horizons for fellow medical practitioners. In the past, sensitive skin treatments as well as conditions that could not be cured, such as oily outside but dry inside, enlarged pores, skin itchiness, papulopustules, baffled me. Now, I realize that these symptoms may be associated with *Demodex*. His findings largely improved our diagnostic accuracy and benefited numerous patients.

Let us not miss the fact that these glorious achievements, clinical research findings, publication of papers, and speeches, are from just one physician who practices in a private primary clinic, not the one in a medical center who can pay full attention to research.

Dr. Huang and I are both dermatologists trained at the Department of Dermatology of National Cheng Kung University Hospital, where Dr. Huang started his training many years earlier than me. My discussions with him regarding various skin problems are always inspiring. I am also highly impressed by his meticulous clinical observation, in-depth research, and rigorous academic attitude. All the more so, as a senior physician, Dr. Huang is not inert to youngsters in the modern world. He keeps close pace with the time and is constantly improving in many aspects, such as managing Facebook communities, producing YouTube videos, shooting promotional materials, and even producing slides. Every time I chat with Dr. Huang, who is both a teacher and a friend to me, and praise his outstanding achievements, he always humbly replies to me, "I still have much to learn from young people." To think this way, how many senior doctors would be willing to tread out of their comfort zone and make changes to catch up with the trend?

Today, Dr. Huang is willing to unsparingly share his clinical experience and research findings through this book in English. It is suitable for the general public and doctors in different departments to obtain a larger picture and detailed mechanisms to enable readers to learn correct concepts through evidence-based data, ensuring the best treatment and care for patients with rosacea. I heartfully recommend this book!

Dean of Jeng-Hsien Lin Dermatology Clinic
Lin Jeng-Hsien

# Foreword 5

My understanding of *Demodex* started with Prof. Lee Yu-Yun's case study. Prof. Lee noticed *Demodex* mites surrounded by granulomatous inflammation in a skin biopsy of a patient whose face showed diffuse papules. This typical case of demodicosis prompted Prof. Lee to initiate a retrospective study on skin pathology. Her findings won the Best Poster Award at the Dermatological Conference in 2007, and her paper was accepted by the Journal of the American Academy of Dermatology in 2009. In the following years after the acceptance, we did not see any cases of demodicosis, and I personally was very much occupied by genetic research on keloids and hereditary skin diseases. The topic of *Demodex* gradually lost my attention.

One day in 2015, Prof. Lee sent me an email inviting me to participate in Dr. Huang's research meeting. After the meeting, Dr. Huang invited me to his place to discuss his methods to examine *Demodex* quantification: superficial needle-scraping (SNS) for pustules and thumbnail-squeezing method (TSM). I can still recall the scene vividly. Mrs. Huang prepared exquisite fruits and snacks, with top-quality Japanese green tea at the side, which made me feel very welcomed. Even more impressive to me was that Dr. Huang had just finished three shifts in his OPD clinic outpatient on that day. Yet, he seemed to have full energy to talk about his interesting clinical observations through countless clinical and microscopic photos, and I wondered about the effort and time he had invested in studying *Demodex*. During the discussion, he even mentioned that he got up in the middle of the night to observe the culture of *Demodex*, which was cultivated using sebum from steatocystoma. As a physician at a medical center, his research perseverance humbled me and won my respect for him.

Among Dr. Huang's many findings, my favorite is the TSM. This method enables us to quantify *Demodex* at skin lesion sites, providing an important reference for disease treatment and follow-up. In addition, this method gives us opportunities to obtain a large number of *Demodex* samples for subsequent research mechanism. I deeply believe that this method will be included in the chapters on rosacea and demodicosis in dermatological textbooks.

I am honored to have the opportunity to participate in Dr. Huang's research journey on rosacea and *Demodex*. I firmly believe that Dr. Huang will make more breakthrough developments in this field in the future.

Professor and Doctor, Department of Dermatology,
National Cheng Kung University Medical School
Chao-Kai Hsu
許釗凱

# Preface

In 2012, it was the first time we had discovered *Demodex* in a case of recurrent papulopustules without diffuse erythema on the face. Prior to that, we knew very little about this parasite that coexists with humans. We only knew from textbooks that *Demodex* was one of the triggers of rosacea. At the time, metronidazole gel and doxycycline were the two common medications to treat rosacea. There was not much experience in the use of other medications, such as β-blockers (propranolol), tacrolimus ointment, and pimecrolimus cream. In the same year, Dr. Chia-Kai Hsu and Prof. Yu-Yun Lee from the Department of Dermatology of National Cheng Kung University Hospital published their findings on the application of carvedilol to treat facial erythema and flushing caused by rosacea. It took years to gain experiences in the treatment of rosacea using pulsed dye laser.

Subsequently, we discovered several patients with *Demodex* overgrowth. Most of them were patients with rosacea, and some had suffered from chronic and recurrent papulopustules. Without an optimal medication option for *Demodex*, we had no choice but to use medications for scabies, benzyl benzoate lotion, and tea tree oil to help some patients fight against the annoying rosacea. In 2017, the anti-*Demodex* and anti-inflammatory medication was finally made available in Taiwan. Since then, it has become easier to treat rosacea, and most patients are satisfied with their treatment outcomes. In the past 10 years, along with the two innovative methods to examine *Demodex*, starting from patients with rosacea that was ineffective to non-anti-*Demodex* treatment, and then comprehensively screening the DMD of patients with rosacea, we have successfully introduced anti-*Demodex* treatments. Meanwhile, an increasingly complex issue emerged. Some patients exhibited acute exacerbation after receiving anti-*Demodex* treatment, rendering the outcomes of this treatment unpredictable and comparable to opening Pandora's box. Fortunately, after a series of research and observations and a comparison of the mechanisms of *Demodex* and its etiology and pathology, we learned that the death of *Demodex* causes a severe skin reaction. Currently, we are capable of screening out these high-risk patients in advance and protecting them from adverse reactions caused by anti-*Demodex* treatment.

In 2017, the global ROSacea COnsensus (ROSCO) panel proposed the diagnosis, classification, and treatments for rosacea based on phenotypes. In 2019, the global ROSCO panel reaffirmed its conclusion announced in 2017 without a further breakthrough in treatment. In 2022, the Taiwanese Dermatological Association also held a ROSCO conference. Unlike the global ROSCO, the conference considered the assessment of *Demodex* and the treatments for rosacea. Although a treatment guideline was published after the meeting, I believe the progress we had made on rosacea since 2017 was far ahead. Therefore, by integrating the research in dermatology, neurology, physiology, circulation, biomedicine, and pharmacology, we speculated that nitric oxide is vital in the development of facial erythema and flushing caused by rosacea. We were fortunate to discover a scavenger to inhibit nitric oxide. Simultaneously, we obtained a better understanding of the effect of botulinum toxin A on neurovascular dysregulation in rosacea. In terms of treatment based on phenotypes proposed by the global ROSCO, we extended its guideline to specific targets in the pathogenesis of trigger factors and proposed pathway-level and target-based treatments. The pathway levels of treatment include (1) anti-*Demodex* treatment to treat rosacea and prevention of flare-ups caused by anti-*Demodex* strategies, (2) treatment of facial erythema and flushing caused by heat and stress and reduction in sympathetic response of the skin, and (3) anti–nitric oxide treatment. Our clinical observations showed that, except for a small number of neurogenic rosacea and flushing related to sleep, our approach is adequate to treat the vast majority of rosacea cases. These observations have resulted in summarizing crucial clinical treatments and descriptions in Taiwan.

Rosacea has attracted the attention of many dermatologists and the public in Taiwan in recent years. One of the significant factors is the advancement in treatment. In the past, through lectures, seminars, health education activities, and social media, many dermatologists and patients with rosacea became aware of this issue and its treatments. Now, we have set out to compose a book on rosacea in Taiwan, covering information for clinical practice and health education to patients with rosacea.

Through the Taiwan ROSCO conference, we got an opportunity to carefully compile the clinical experience, statistical data, research findings we have published over the past 10 years, and stories of our patients with rosacea into a book. This book, with detailed accounts of our thought processes and procedures for rosacea diagnosis and treatment, partially fills the gap between the most advanced clinical progress and the global ROSCO (2019) and is particularly useful because of the comprehensive coverage of our clinical development. Ocular rosacea is one of the important rosacea subtypes. Associate Professor Yeh Lung-Kun is the chief physician in the corneal division at the Department of Ophthalmology of Linkou Chang Gung Memorial Hospital. He has a strong academic background and eminent publications over 100. He has in-depth research and clinical experience on *Demodex* infection and rosacea in the eye. In the consensus conference held by the Taiwanese Dermatological Association, Yeh was invited to give a keynote speech. We are honored to invite him to compose the chapter on ocular rosacea in this book, which enriches and complements this book.

In 2015, because of the negative connotations, Prof. Lee Yu-Yun proposed renaming the translated name of rosacea in mandarin from "wine dregs nose" to "rose spot." In the ROSCO conference (2022) held by the Taiwanese Dermatological Association, the proposal was approved by the majority of the board members. I chose the formal name, rosacea, at most of the instances in this book and the old name, rosacea, at certain instances to ensure consistent rhetoric. I want to convey my gratitude to Prof. Yu-Yun Lee, Prof. Chao-Kai Hsu, and senior experts at the Department of Dermatology of National Cheng Kung University Hospital, who educated and supported me during the course.

# Contents

# 1

# About Rosacea

## 1.1 Introduction to the disease

### 1.1.1 *Preface*

As a chronic inflammatory facial disease, rosacea has common symptoms such as erythema, flushing, papules, pustules, or telangiectasis, with burning sensation and dry skin. Patients with severe conditions have a hypertrophied nose (Figure 1).[1] Many patients with rosacea may find their quality of life affected because of the change in their facial appearance, which leads to psychological burden and makes them prone to anxiety and depression.[2,3] The cause of rosacea is still unclear. Recent research shows that the primary causes of rosacea include genetic predisposition, abnormal immune responses, and abnormal neurovascular responses.[4]

The Chinese disease name of rosacea is "wine dregs nose or alcoholic nose," originally meant rosy and got its name from the feature of erythema. Because some patients develop facial redness, nose swelling, or rhinophyma, this disease is misrelated to chronic alcohol consumption. The Chinese nickname for rosacea can mislead people to believe that this disease is related to alcohol consumption. In fact, only about half of patients with rosacea are found with a cause related to alcohol. In view of negative connotation associated with rosacea, Prof. Yu-Yun Lee from the Department of Dermatology of National Cheng Kung University Hospital in 2005 published an article in *Dermatologica Sinica*, "Rosacea: clinical

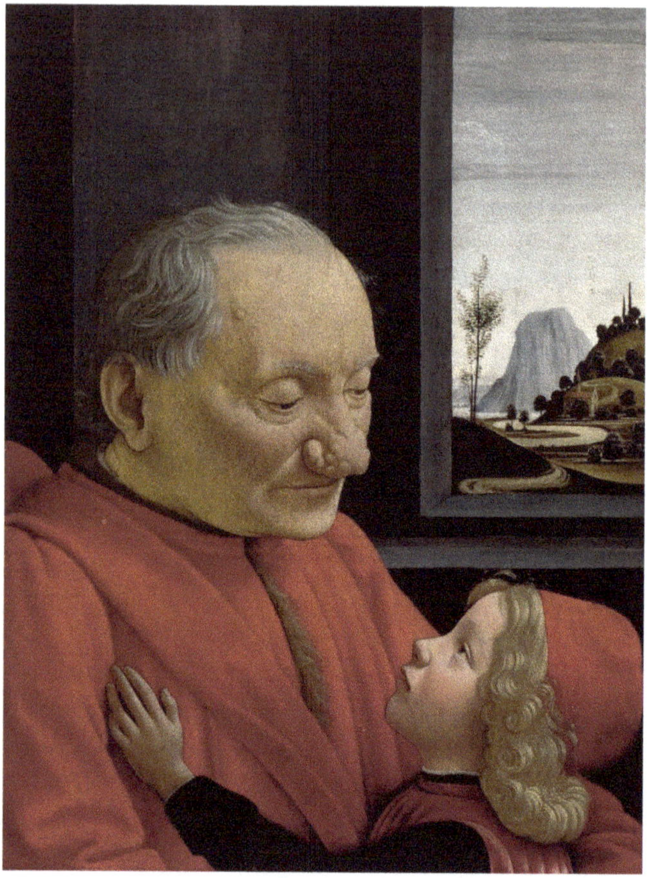

**Figure 1.** *An Old Man with His Grandson*, painted by **Domenico Ghirlandaio** (circa 1490). The elderly man demonstrates nasal hypertrophy and facial erythema, clinical features consistent with rhinophyma associated with rosacea. Source: Wikipedia.

aspects, pathogenesis and treatment," to formally use the term "rose spot" instead of "wine dregs nose" (in Chinese), first time in Taiwan.

In 2015, in the first ROSCO conference organized by the Taiwanese Dermatology Association, Prof. Yu-Yun Lee first proposed the formal name of Chinese disease name of rosacea to "rosacea." Since then, over the years many doctors and public organizations have been using the term "rosacea" over "alcoholic nose." In 2022, in the ROSCO conference by the Taiwanese Dermatology Association, the new name was approved by the majority of the committee members. Because of the long-term use of the accustomed nickname, in certain fields, authors prefer to use both the formal name and the nickname, for example, rosacea in the eye.

Rosacea is a common skin disease that affects 5%–10% of people. The prevalence rate is as high as 12.3% in Germany and 5.0% in Russia.[5] There is no clear data on the prevalence of rosacea in Taiwan, but it is estimated at 5%–10%. In Huang Hui-Peng Dermatology Clinic, in the recent 5 years, patients with rosacea have accounted for approximately 10% of all patients seen. The disease is more prevalent in females at the age of 30–60 years. In recent years, it is more common in younger patients. From 2002 to 2017, although the diagnostic criteria for rosacea were relatively broad, according to an article by Prof. Yu-Yun Lee from the Department of Dermatology of National Cheng Kung University Hospital in 2004, only about 40% of the patients with rosacea were diagnosed correctly for the first time. Many of these patients were misdiagnosed with other skin diseases, such as eczema, skin allergies, seborrheic dermatitis, contact dermatitis, acne, and lupus erythematosus. Because the 2017 ROSCO panel proposed phenotype-based classification and treatment for rosacea, the diagnostic criteria have become strict. Theoretically, there should have been fewer patients meeting the criteria; however, the number of patients receiving rosacea diagnosis has been increasing. Fortunately, patients with rosacea who used steroids long-term because of misdiagnosis has become rare. This should be attributed to the fact that dermatologists and patients generally pay attention to rosacea.

In the past, rosacea was more common in females with white complexion. Now, we have realized that rosacea can also be found in those with dark skin. These cases are harder to notice in the clinic because the skin color may conceal the clinical signs. Since the proposal of phenotype-based treatment in 2017, which provides clinical doctors a reference for treatment and has improved treatment outcomes substantially, many dermatologists in Taiwan have made efforts in this approach and obtained remarkable results.

The mainstream treatment for rosacea is phenotype-based, which appears perfect in classification yet is considered unorganized. For example, treatment recommendations for papulopustules include five to six options: metronidazole gel/cream, azelaic acid, topical ivermectin, doxycycline, isotretinoin, or even relatively uncommon pimecrolimus, raising the question of how to make a clinical decision. There are recommended medicines for patients with minor, moderate, and severe conditions, but a pathogenesis-based approach has not been developed. Treatment for each patient is randomly determined by chance, like rolling a dice. Considering the example of topical ivermectin, patients likely exhibit an exacerbation rate at the likelihood of 1.4%, 5.4%, 24%, 38%, 75%, to 100% according to features of patients and treatment combinations. Without a system providing guidelines to match treatment and disease subtypes, treatment outcomes can be highly unpredictable. The same situation can apply to erythema and flushing. Outcomes are expectable for those treatments whose mechanisms are clear. For those with unclear mechanisms, we would like to predict the treatment success rate and screen out those with high risks to the treatment.

This book mainly focuses on clinical application alongside academic and patient health education. Besides phenotype-based treatment, many chapters are dedicated to pathway-level and targeted treatment, particularly for those confined to the three pathway levels: *Demodex*, heat, and stress, with a preliminary assessment that shows favorable indications. By controlling *Demodex*, heat, and stress, disease activity and flares may be minimized. By taking the initiative, I hope I will attract more people's attention to rosacea. I also hope that we will be able to control and eradicate rosacea someday.

## 1.2 Diagnosis

### 1.2.1 *Differential diagnosis of rosacea*

According to the classification from the National Rosacea Society (NRS) in the US in 2002, there are four subtypes of rosacea: erythematotelangiectatic rosacea (ETR), papulopustular rosacea (PPR), phymatous rosacea, and ocular rosacea. The diagnostic criteria for rosacea cover any one or more of the four features: facial flushing, persistent erythema, papulopustule, and telangiectasis.[1] In the global ROSacea COnsensus (ROSCO) project (2017), the panel updated the diagnosis, classification, and treatment of rosacea. A diagnosis of rosacea is made using one diagnostic feature or two or more major features (Table 1).[6] The same year, the NRS

**Table 1.** Diagnostic features, major features, and minor or secondary features of rosacea

| **Diagnostic features (≥75% consensus)** | **Major features (≥50% agreement)** | **Minor features (≥75% consensus)** |
|---|---|---|
| Persistent centrofacial erythema associated with periodic intensification by potential trigger factors | Flushing/transient centrofacial erythema | Burning sensation of the skin |
| Phymatous changes | Inflammatory papules and pustules | Stinging sensation of the skin |
| | Telangiectasia | Edema |
| | Ocular manifestations<br>Lid margin telangiectasis<br>Blepharitis<br>Keratitis/conjunctivitis/sclerokeratitis | Dry sensation of the skin |

Reference: *Br J Dermatol.* 2017;176(2):431–438.

**Table 2.** Clinical features of rosacea

| **Diagnostic features*** | **Major features**† | **Minor features** |
|---|---|---|
| Fixed centrofacial erythema in a characteristic pattern that may periodically intensify<br>Phymatous changes | • Flushing,<br>• Papules and pustules,<br>• Telangiectasia,<br>• Ocular manifestations:<br>• Lid margin telangiectasia,<br>• Interpalpebral conjunctival Injection,<br>• Spade-shaped infiltrates in the cornea,<br>• Scleritis and sclerokeratitis | • Burning sensation<br>• Stinging sensation<br>• Edema<br>• Dryness<br>• Ocular manifestations<br>• "Honey crust" and collarette accumulation at the base of the lashes<br>• Irregularity of the lid margin<br>• Evaporative tear dysfunction (rapid tear breakup time) |

Note: *These features by themselves are diagnostic of rosacea.
†Two or more major features may be considered diagnostic.
Reference: *J Am Acad Dermatol.* 2018;78(1):148–155.

in the US embraced the criteria and indicated that the diagnosis of rosacea may be considered once a patient exhibits two or more major features.[7] The ROSCO (2019) extended the guidelines released in the ROSCO (2017). To assist diagnosis and evaluation, the 2019 ROSCO panel provided complementary descriptions regarding skin features.[8]

One of two phenotype-based diagnostic features can be used to diagnose rosacea, which are (1) fixed centrofacial erythema in a characteristic pattern that may periodically intensify (Figure 2) and (2) phymatous changes. Fixed centrofacial erythema may periodically intensify according to the presence of trigger factors.[8] Characteristic pattern refers to the convex surface areas, such as the cheek, forehead, nose, and chin.[1] The area of erythema varies, though the author believes that the involvement of bilateral cheeks can ensure a more accurate diagnosis. In some cases, neurogenic rosacea affects the peripheral areas of the cheek,[9] even the upper eyelids and the ears (Figure 3). Phymatous changes refer to facial skin thickening led by skin fibrosis and/or sebaceous hyperplasia. The nose is the most commonly affected site; once affected, it may change to a bulbous appearance.[8] Rhinophyma may or may not be concomitant with inflammation or facial erythema (Figure 4).

For cases with fixed centrofacial erythema, the following conditions need to be ruled out: contact dermatitis caused by topical medicines, retinoic acid, or glycolic acid peeling (Figure 5A); long-term use of topical steroid; erythema caused by treatment using energy-based devices (Figure 5B); dermatomyositis; systemic lupus erythematosus; and photodermatitis.

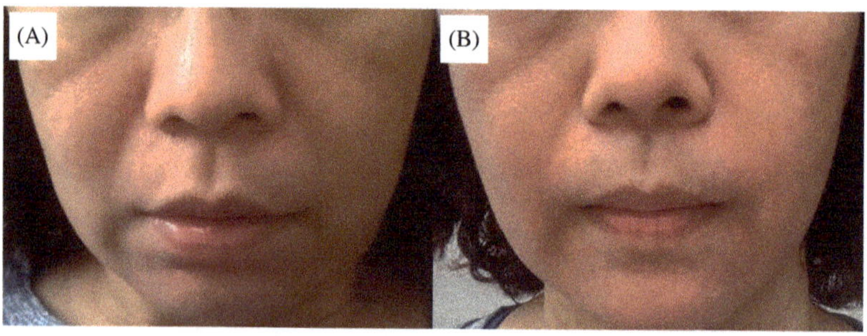


**Figure 2.** Fixed centrofacial erythema in a characteristic pattern (A) that becomes more noticeable after exercise (B), which is a diagnostic feature of rosacea.

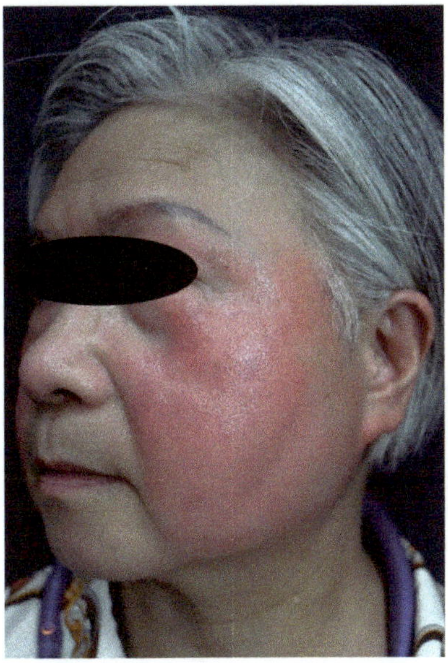

**Figure 3.** Neurogenic rosacea affects the peripheral areas of the cheek, lower jaws, and even the upper eyelids and ears.

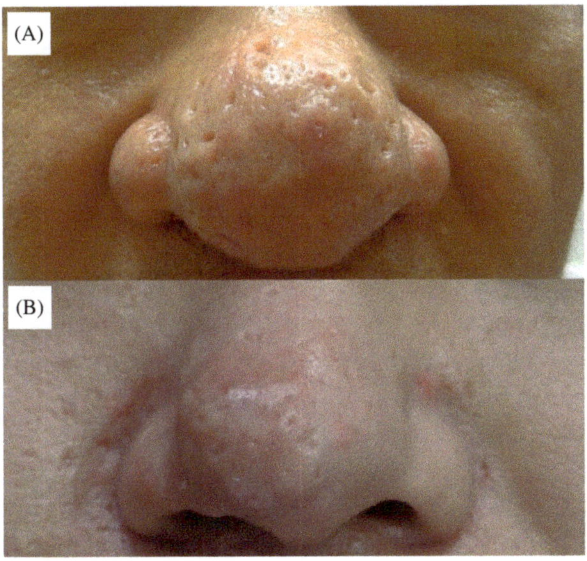

**Figure 4.** Rhinophyma, thickening of the nose to a bulbous appearance due to fibrosis and sebaceous hyperplasia (A); rhinophyma without accompanying erythema on the face (B).

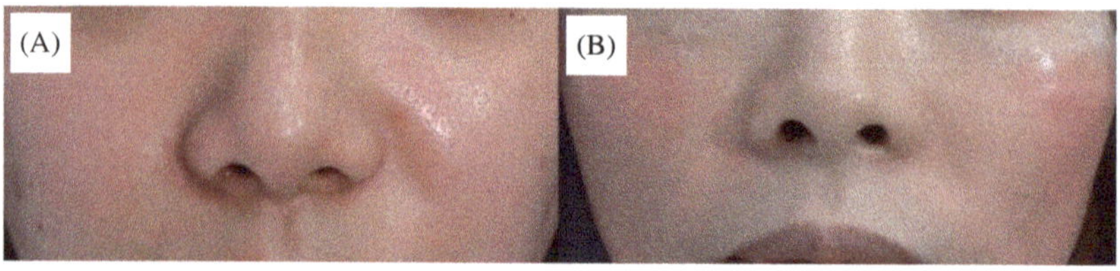


**Figure 5.** Contact dermatitis. Facial erythema caused by topical medicine, adapalene gel (A); erythema caused by the treatment using 1064-nm picolaser (B).

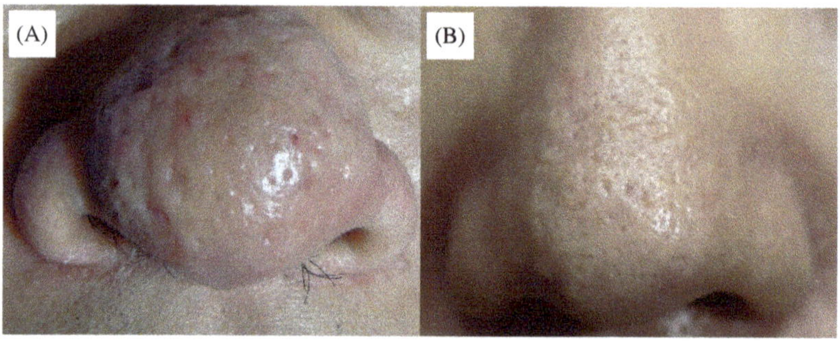


**Figure 6.** The protruding and thickening of the nose caused by rhinophyma (A) and acne (B) are different. The latter are scars following cystic acne, without sebaceous hyperplasia.

Atopic dermatitis on the face often develops lichenification. Seborrheic dermatitis can be differentiated by the appearance of oily and flaky light-yellow areas in the eyebrow and creases at the base of the nose, behind the ears, and the external auditory meatus. Patients with rosacea are commonly found with seborrheic dermatitis. When there is a case presenting with facial erythema, demodicosis need not be suspected right away. Redness is not the primary symptom of demodicosis. Many diseases can lead to facial erythema, and rosacea accounts for a proportion. The protruding and thickening seen in noninflammatory rhinophyma and acne are different. The latter are scars after cystic acne, without sebaceous hyperplasia (Figure 6).

In the 2017 global ROSCO project, in addition to the above two diagnostic features, there are four major features: flushing, papules and pustules, telangiectasia, and ocular manifestations. The first three features are in the centrofacial area, with a bilateral distribution. The major features garnered ≥50% consensus in the panel, and the diagnostic features gained ≥75% consensus (Table 1). Following the global ROSCO, in the same year, the American NRS also adopted the phenotype-based diagnostic criteria, with an additional note that two or more major features may be considered diagnostic.[7] Based on clinical experience, I also agree that a diagnosis of rosacea based on two or even more major features is less accurate than one diagnostic feature.

Facial flushing in rosacea is transient erythema in the centrofacial area, which may combine sensations of warmth, heat, burning, and/or stinging.[8] Based on my clinical observations, upon asking patients to perform arithmetic tasks, the flushing changes like a rising tide, with the color getting redder and the affected area expanding. The flushing may disappear in a few seconds and reoccur in cyclic manner. In some cases, the flushing prolongs for more than 10 minutes in conditions such as after long-duration exercise. There are many factors that trigger rosacea flushing, such as heat (including hot drinks, whole-body heating, and local face heat), emotions, stress, exercise, alcohol, and spicy food. Emotional flushing/blushing appears in the centrofacial area, and both negative and positive emotions, such as images of erotica or mutilation, can trigger sympathetic neurovascular responses.[10,11]

Normal healthy people can develop very minor and almost unnoticeable facial flushing even when they encounter arithmetic tests. Patients with rosacea have augmented emotional flushing. According to studies, there may be dozens of physical conditions and diseases that can trigger flushing, yet most flushing in these conditions is not limited to the center of the face.[10,12] Flushing caused by menopause is a sudden feeling of warmth in the upper body, and the cause is hypoestrogenism resulting in hypersensitivity of the hypothalamus thermal center to the change of body temperature. The course includes a flush of heat for 30 seconds and then sweating for 30 seconds, sometimes flushing combined.[13]

Papules and pustules of rosacea are usually centrofacial, and some may be larger and deeper.[8] Papulopustules caused by some diseases other than rosacea can also be centrofacial. Pustular demodicosis, with a high *Demodex* mite density (DMD), is usually centrofacial without a significant background of erythema with an asymmetrical distribution. In acne vulgaris, white-headed or black-headed comedones can be found.

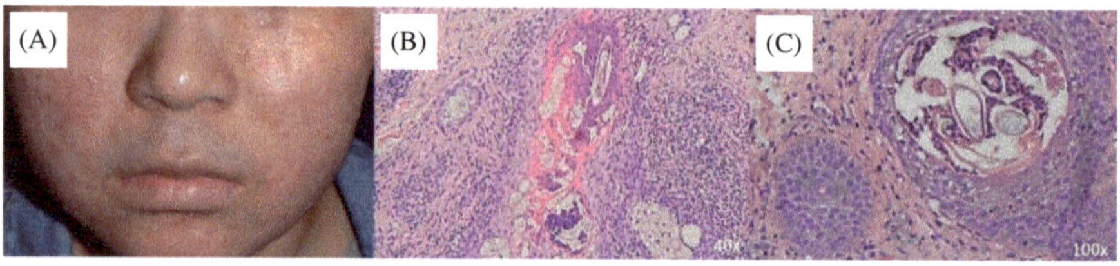


**Figure 7.** Eosinophilic pustular folliculitis combined with demodicosis. A 24-year-old female who has had pruritic red papules and nodules on her face for 2 years (A). Histopathology examination showed a folliculocentric eosinophil-rich infiltrate with infundibular pustules containing multiple *Demodex* mites (B, C) (hematoxylin and eosin staining, x40 and x400), and *Demodex* evaluation showed 225 mites/cm$^2$.

References: Huang HP, Hsu CK, Chao SC, Yang CC, Chen GS, Lin CH, Huang. CM, Lee JY. Eosinophilic pustular folliculitis associated with *Demodex* overgrowth or demodicosis on the face — A report of five cases. *Dermatol Sin* 2021; 39:132–6.

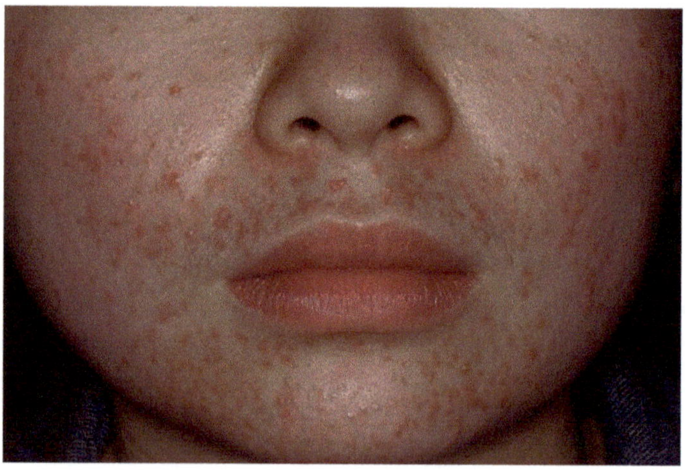

**Figure 8.** Monomorphous papulopustules are the characteristic feature of Pityrosporum folliculitis. (Thanks to the photo provider, Dr. Lo Chi-Shou)

Eosinophilic pustular folliculitis (EPF) (Figure 7) and *Pityrosporum* folliculitis (Figure 8) can also sometimes cause centrofacial papulopustules, but each has its own features. Classic EPF, Ofuji's disease, exhibits annular configuration and causes postinflammatory hyperpigmentation; *Pityrosporum* folliculitis develops monomorphous papules.

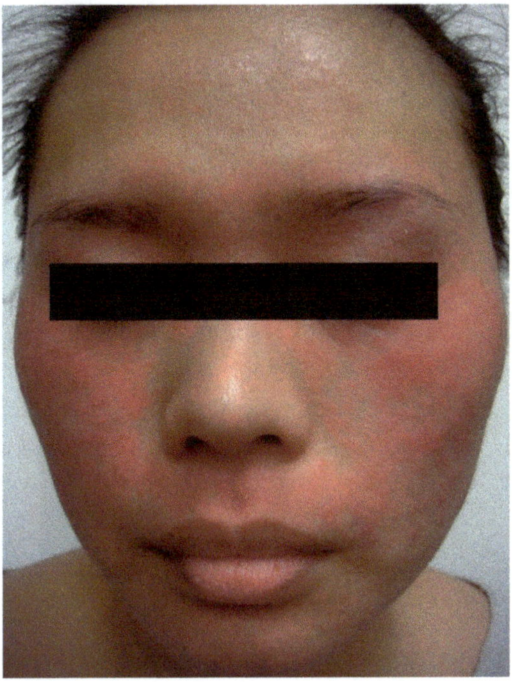

**Figure 9.** Tinea faciei manifested as scaly erythema and small pustules on the face with an annular active edge on the forehead. KOH smear showed branching septate hyphae.

Papulopustules caused by perioral dermatitis are mainly found around the mouth or nose. A few cases of tinea faciei also exhibit facial erythema and pustules (Figure 9). According to the 2019 global ROSCO project, telangiectasia of rosacea refers to visible vessels in the centrofacial area, including but not limited to the alar area (Figure 10A).[8] We conducted a survey of facial telangiectasis in 81 young Taiwanese women aged 14–40 years. The presence of facial telangiectasis in the lower cheek and perinasal and alar folds was 89% in 18 patients with rosacea, 68% in 38 patients with acne, and 76% in 25 patients with other nonfacial conditions and healthy controls. Therefore, if telangiectasia in the lower cheeks and perinasal and alar folds have been present since childhood (Figure 10B), the author suggests not considering these signs as a major feature of rosacea.

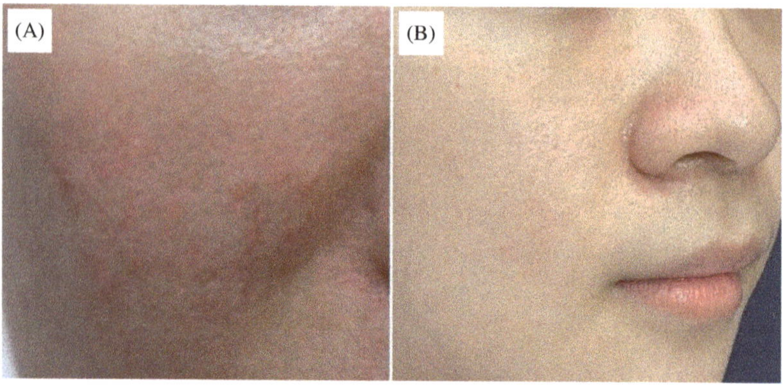

**Figure 10.** A patient with rosacea and central facial erythema and flushing had telangiectasis in the paranasal folds and the area under the nose and the cheek (A). A 22-year-old healthy female had visible capillaries in the paranasal folds and the lower cheek (B).

### 1.2.2 *Differential diagnosis of demodicosis and rosacea*

The differential diagnosis of demodicosis and rosacea is complicated. *Demodex* is one of the trigger factors for rosacea. According to previous studies, the density of *Demodex* in patients with rosacea is higher than that in healthy control groups.[14–18] Methods to examine *Demodex* in previous reports include the standardized skin surface biopsy (SSSB),[14] two consecutive standardized skin surface biopsies (SSSB1 + 2),[15] the thumbnail-squeezing method (TSM),[16] the superficial needle-scraping (SNS) for pustules, and[17] reflectance confocal microscopy.[18] The TSM and SNS were published by Dr. Huang Hui-Peng and Prof. Lee Yu-Yun and Prof. Hsu Chao-Kai at National Cheng Kung University Hospital.[15,16] According to the statistics of patients with papulopustular rosacea (PPR) and ETR examined using the TSM, the sensitivity was 92% and specificity is 90% at the cutoff value of >11 *Demodex* mites/cm$^2$. These cases all presented with fixed centrofacial erythema. Based on the confocal microscopy analysis, the sensitivity was 82% and the specificity was 80%, with the cutoff value of >0.17 mites per follicle for distinguishing between demodicosis and normal skin.

According to the results of these two studies, 82%–92% of patients have high DMDs.[16,18]

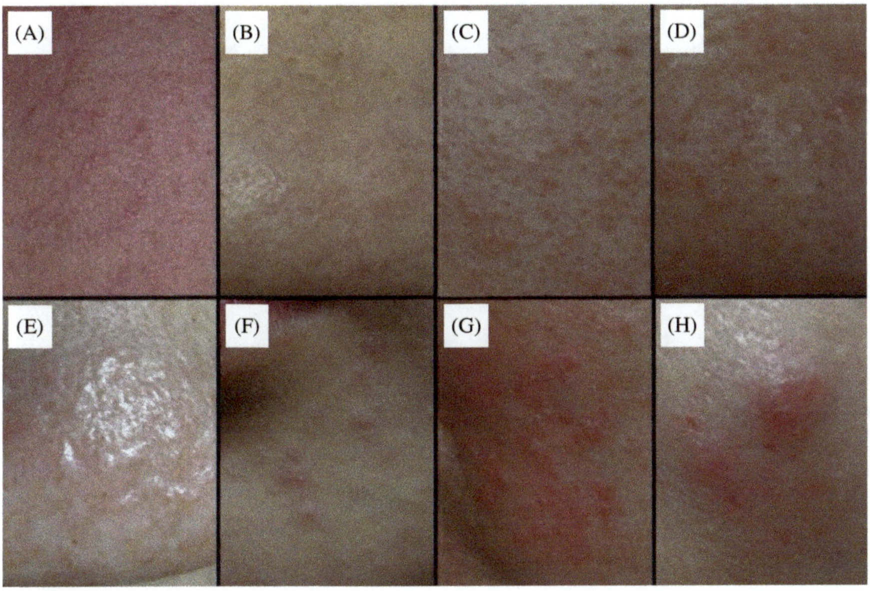


**Figure 11.** In papulopustular demodicosis, patients with papules only can have lesions of the size of a pinpoint, pinhead, or plaques if multiple lesions are fused together (A–E); those with papulopustules can have lesions of the size of a pinpoint, pinhead, or nodulocysts (F–H).

According to the classification by Dr. Huang Hui-Peng, the clinical manifestations of demodicosis include papulopustular type (Figure 11) and nonpapulopustular type (Figure 12). The former can be papules only or papulopustules. Patients with papules may only have skin lesions as small as a pinpoint, pinhead, or plaques if multiple lesions are fused together. Those with papulopustules may have skin lesions as large as a pinpoint, pinhead, or nodulocysts (Figure 9). Patients with nonpapulopustular demodicosis may develop large pores and white follicular plugs or scales. Clinical manifestations have several variations: large tan-colored pores formed by enlarged pores, orange skin-like appearance, protruding white spicule-like follicle scales with frosted or sandpaper-like appearance, and the coexistence of enlarged pores and white follicle plugs with nutmeg grater appearance (Figure 12). Some patients with rosacea combined with high DMD may show clinical signs of demodicosis, such as papulopustules, enlarged pores, and white follicle plugs, whereas others

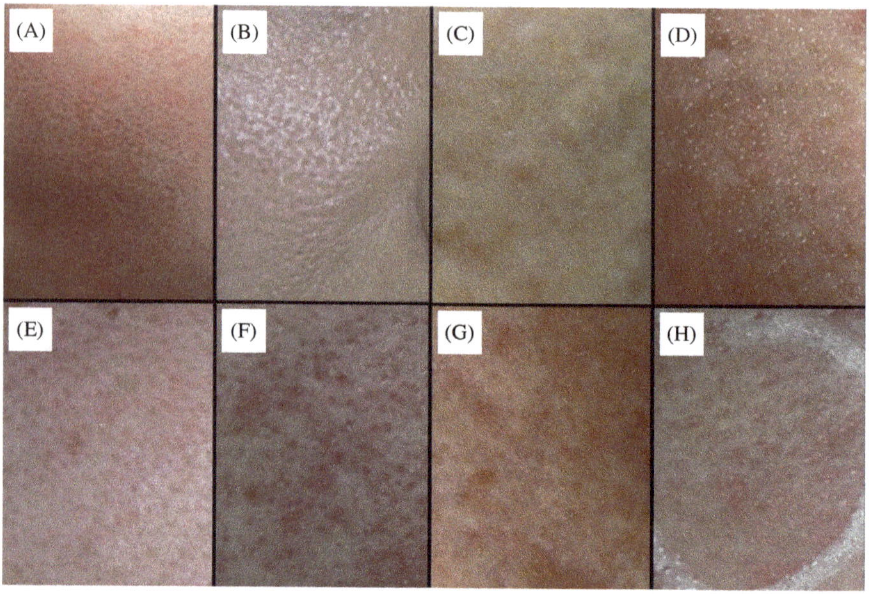


**Figure 12.** Patients with nonpapulopustular demodicosis may develop large pores and follicular plugs or scales. Clinical manifestations may be large tan-colored pores (A) formed by large pores or orange skin-like appearance (B). In addition, the clinical manifestations may be protruding follicular plugs or scales with frosted appearance (C) or sandpaper-like appearance (D) defined by granularity. Furthermore, large pores and white follicular plugs or scales may also coexist, with nutmeg grater-like appearance (E, F, G, and H).

have no clinical signs. In a study on the SNS, 7 of 40 patients with PPR were found with no *Demodex* in their pustules.[17] Thus, papulopustules in patients with rosacea can be a manifestation of demodicosis itself or a feature of rosacea. Enlarged pores and white follicle plugs should be regarded as characteristics formed by the development of demodicosis itself. Those with no signs of demodicosis should be regarded with *Demodex* overgrowth (Figure 13).

According to the review by Dr. Chen Wen-Jie et al., demodicosis can be classified into primary demodicosis and secondary demodicosis.[19]

The latter often combines general or partial immune insufficiency. There are three criteria for the diagnosis of primary demodicosis: (1) no previous or simultaneous inflammatory disease, such as acne, rosacea, or

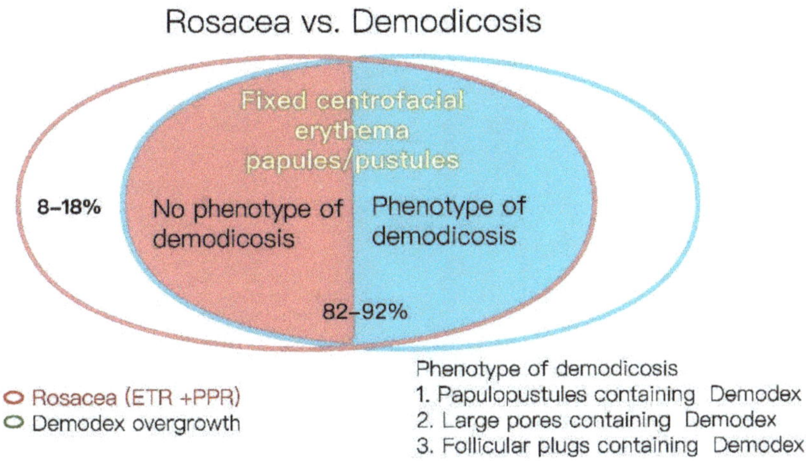


**Figure 13.** For patients with rosacea presenting with persistent centrofacial erythema that may periodically intensify (ETR) or papulopustules (PPR), results obtained through the confocal microscope evaluation and the thumbnail-squeezing method show that the percentage of patients with rosacea having high *Demodex* density ranges from 82% to 92%. Some of the patients having high *Demodex* density were found with clinical features of demodicosis, and the others had no such features. ETR: erythematotelangiectatic rosacea; PPR: papulopustular rosacea.

perioral dermatitis; (2) abnormal *Demodex* overgrowth in the in vivo sample from a skin lesion; (3) the eradication of the disease relies on oral or topical acaricides rather than just antibiotics with anti-inflammatory effects, such as tetracycline, doxycycline, or macrolides.[19] It is not appropriate to classify patients with rosacea and demodicosis skin lesions into the group of secondary demodicosis, as some of the patients with demodicosis developed diagnostic or major features of rosacea after some time of follow-up.

As noted in our published paper, patients' large pores and follicular plugs or scales disappeared or were significantly improved after topical antiparasitic drugs were administered for 1–3 months. For most patients, their papulopustules disappeared or were significantly improved, but their fixed centrofacial erythema did not disappear completely.[20] Based on therapeutic outcomes, we can infer that *Demodex* can lead to or worsen facial erythema and papulopustules. Moreover, antiparasitic drugs are effective in treating patients with rosacea and excessive *Demodex*.

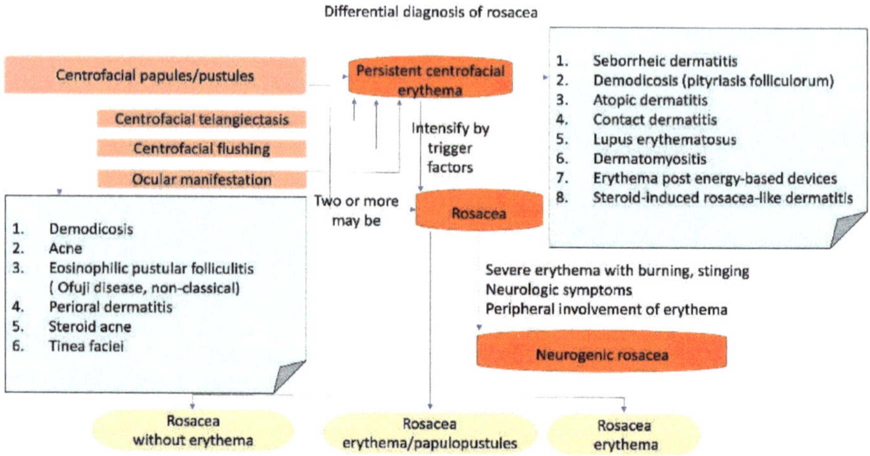


**Figure 14.** Summary of diagnosis and differential diagnosis of rosacea. Either persistent centrofacial erythema that is exacerbated by trigger factors or rhinophyma can be adequate for the diagnosis of rosacea. Patients with rosacea along with severe erythema and burning or stinging sensation or with peripheral face involvement and neurological symptoms are diagnosed with neurogenic rosacea. Those with two or more of the following major features may be diagnosed with rosacea: centrofacial papulopustules, centrofacial flushing, telangiectasia, and ocular manifestations. Differential diagnosis of many diseases is required for persistent centrofacial erythema and papulopustules.

Rosacea is a disease with unclear cause, and its diagnosis on some level relies on ruling out other diseases, which makes its diagnosis complicated. In this book, we summarize the differential diagnosis in Figure 14. According to the phenotype-based treatment guidelines, even for patients exhibiting one major feature, treatment should be given according to symptom severity.

Patients exhibiting two or more major features can be regarded as rosacea cases; however, treatment should be given according to symptom severity. Additionally, patients should be followed up to check whether they develop fixed centrofacial erythema (which is deemed as a diagnostic feature). It is not recommended to jump to the conclusion that *Demodex* overgrowth is the case. In our study on rosacea, 92% of the patients were found with high *Demodex* density; however, these cases were patients with ETR and PPR with fixed centrofacial erythema and cyclic exacerbation and are different from those whose diagnosis is based on two or more major features.[16,17,20,21] Some patients with acne are diagnosed with rosacea because the acne are misrecognized as papulopustules. Symptoms such as minor capillary patterns in the paranasal folds or lower cheek can hardly meet the criteria for rosacea diagnosis. Even with misdiagnosis, treatment is unnecessary for those with minor symptoms. For patients with acne and mild facial redness, the author suggests arithmetic tasks for stress-induced flushing reactions to aid in confirming the diagnosis of rosacea.

In recent years, through the health education activities of the Taiwanese Dermatological Association and related organizations, with the circulation of information in the media, public awareness and attention on rosacea have substantially increased. It is increasingly important for dermatologists to correctly diagnose a rosacea case and differentiate such a case from other diseases. Dermatologists have opportunities to provide improved care for patients with rosacea. Through inquiry and *Demodex* examination, we can help patients with rosacea find out any existing trigger factors, such as *Demodex*, heat, depression, anxiety, excessive cosmetic procedures, antihypertensive drugs, inappropriate cleaning and care, and sun exposure. A comprehensive analysis can lead to a treatment plan covering etiological-level treatment and symptom treatment.

### 1.2.3 *Common differential diagnoses*

Is facial erythema a phenotype of *Demodex*?

The answer is no. Accurate diagnosis is the key to effective treatment. Those with rosacea erythema that is centrofacially persistent in the convex surface and that worsens with exacerbating factors such as emotional changes and heat stimulation need to be considered with *Demodex* overgrowth. For other diseases with centrofacial erythema, it is necessary to assess the cause instead of recommending *Demodex* test for patients. See below for case photos.

#### 1.2.3.1 *Seborrheic dermatitis*

The patient in Figure 15 shows classic erythema symptoms, including yellowish greasy scales in the areas around the eyebrow, cheek, paranasal groove, and around the corners of the mouth, with skin rashes extending to the neck.

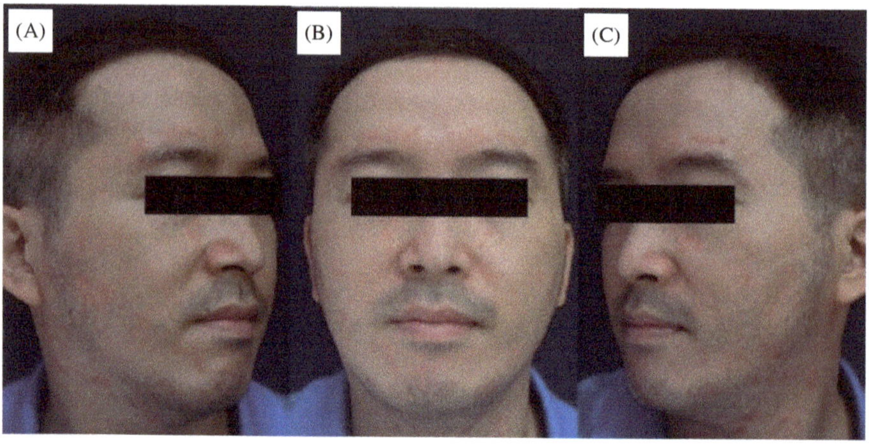


**Figure 15.** Seborrheic dermatitis features facial erythema in the areas around the eyebrow, cheek, paranasal groove, and the corners of the mouth, with noticeable yellowish greasy scales. The patient also shows skin rashes around the ears and lower jaw.

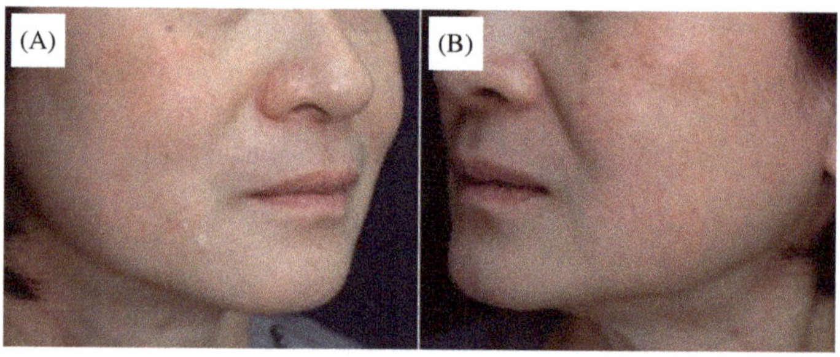


**Figure 16.** Facial erythema, telangiectasia, and skin atrophy caused by topical steroids.

### 1.2.3.2 *Steroid-induced dermatitis*

The patient in Figure 16 has facial itching caused by long-term application of topical steroids. Later, she developed facial erythema, hypersensitivity, telangiectasia, and skin atrophy. Doctors at other clinics prescribed her with drugs for rosacea. However, we noticed that her facial erythema was mainly located at her lateral cheeks, and she did not show flushing exacerbation during arithmetic tasks or emotional changes. Her symptoms were caused by typical dermatitis resulting from topical steroids, which were very similar to the symptoms of rosacea but not caused by rosacea.

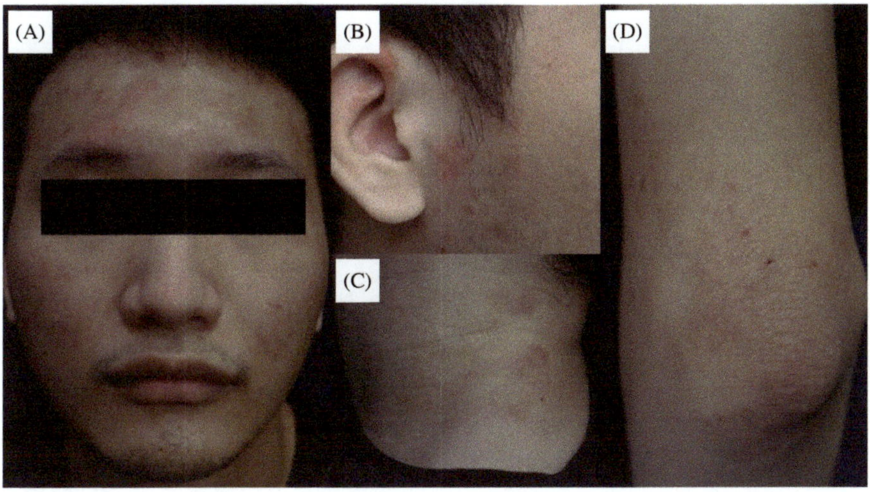


**Figure 17.** Atopic dermatitis manifests with (A) facial erythema, lichenification, and noticeable skin lines. These rashes also appear (B) on and in front of the ear, (C) on the neck, and (D) on the elbow.

### 1.2.3.3 *Atopic dermatitis*

Atopic dermatitis on the face often develops lichenification with noticeable hyperpigmentation, thickening of skin, exaggerated skin lines, and cheilitis as well as a circle of whiteness around the lips. Chronic eczema on the neck, ears, and the flexor sides of four extremities (Figure 17).

### 1.2.3.4 *Dermatomyositis*

The characteristic skin features of dermatomyositis (Figure 18) are heliotrope sign and Gottron papules. Heliotrope sign indicates a violaceous-to-dusky erythema involving the periorbital regions and often on the forehead and behind the ears. Gottron papules are erythematous or violaceous papules or nodules on the joints of hands.[22]

### 1.2.3.5 *Systemic lupus erythematosus*

Discoid lupus erythematosus manifests with discoid, atrophic, and crusted erythema with telangiectasis on the face (Figure 19).

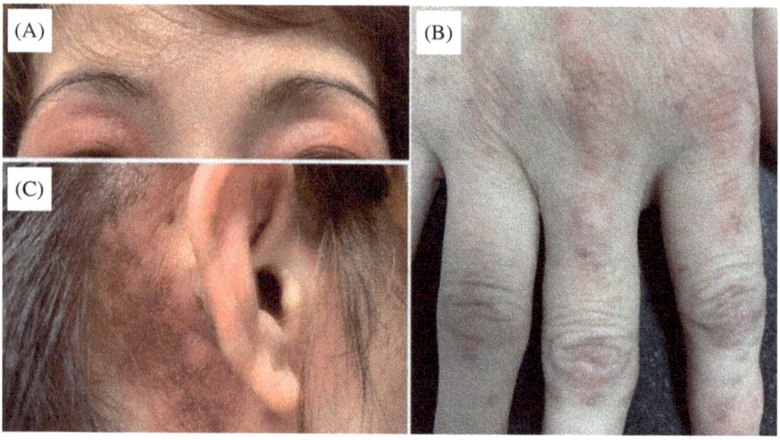


**Figure 18.** Dermatomyositis with (A) facial erythema and heliotrope sign on the eyelids, (B) dusky erythema behind the ears, and (C) Gottron papules on the dorsum of fingers.

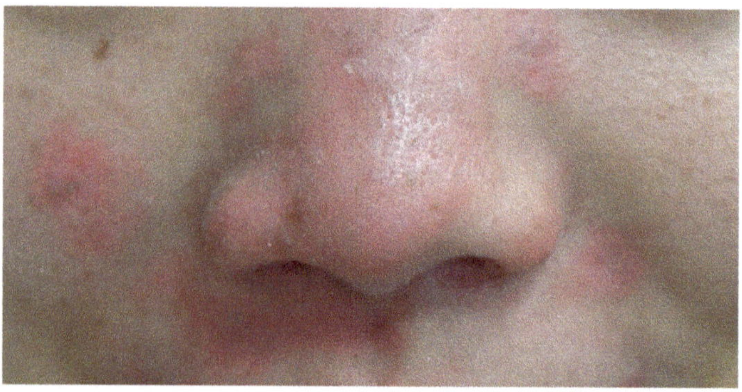

**Figure 19.** Lupus erythematosus with discoid, atrophic, and crusted erythema on the face.

### 1.2.3.6 *Sensitive skin*

Sensitive skin is not a diagnostic term; it refers to a skin condition that has lower tolerance to skincare and cosmetic products. Clinical signs of sensitive skin include stinging, itching, and burning sensations, combined with noticeable skin changes, such as erythema, dryness, scaling, peeling, plaques, and swelling. Sensitive skin is not limited to facial skin. It is also common in the eyelid, armpit, and genitalia. Diseases related to sensitive skin include rosacea, demodicosis, seborrheic dermatitis, atopic dermatitis, irritant contact dermatitis, allergic contact dermatitis, dermatitis caused by treatment using energy-based devices, dermatitis caused by topical steroids, skin dryness, eczema, and photodermatitis. The cause of the disease needs to be assessed based on differential diagnosis carefully conducted by dermatologists. Principles for general skin care include use of soap-free face wash, nonirritating moisturizers, and sunscreen products.

## 1.3 Etiopathology

### 1.3.1 *Multifactorial etiology and pathological mechanism*

Rosacea is a multifactorial disease, and its physiopathological mechanism is still under study. The pathogenesis includes genetic predisposition, dysregulation of immune response, dysregulation of neurovascular response, and other non-neuronal vascular response including vascular adhesion molecules and vascular endothelial growth factor (VEGF) (Figure 20).[23,24] Dysregulation of neurovascular response involves afferent sensory nerve, skin sympathetic nerve, and nitric oxide.[25,26] The trigger factors include ultraviolet (UV) rays, *Demodex* and microbes, stress, emotional changes, heat irritation, exercise, and food, particularly alcohol and spicy food.

Dysregulation of the immune response involves innate immunity and adaptive immunity. *Demodex* and UV irradiation induce rosacea through the activation of the innate immune response. *Demodex* and UV rays induce TLR-2 expression. TLR-2 activates KLK-5 (serine protease) in keratinocytes. KLK-5 cleaves antimicrobial peptides (cathelicidin) into the active form, LL-37. LL-37 induces inflammatory responses, telangiectasis, and angiogenesis in the rosacea. LL-37 can also facilitate the degranulation of mast cells, enhancing matrix metalloproteinase-1 (MMP-1), MMP-9, and IL-6 expression. The precursor of KLK-5 can also transform into KLK-5 under the effect of MMPs. Meanwhile, mast cells at the lesion site increase and get activated by LL-37. In this course, neutrophils, macrophages, and CD4+ cells are activated, thereby releasing more cytokines and MMPs. MMPs also lead to an increase in KLK-5. The increase in the TLR-2 level also induces proinflammatory response.[23,24]

The number of T cells such as Th1 and Th17 at lesion sites is more than that in a normal condition. TH17 secretes IL-17. Through VEGF,

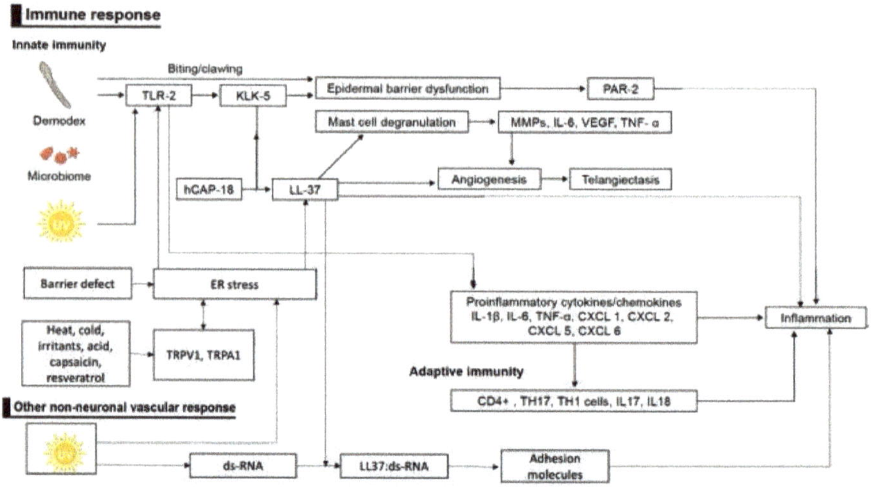


**Figure 20.** The possible mechanisms of innate and adaptive immunity and adhesion molecules in rosacea. TLR-2 is activated by *Demodex*, microbiome, and UVB. Subsequently, TLR-2 activates KLK-5 and increases the expression of proinflammatory cytokines and chemokines. LL-37 activation by either KLK-5 or PAR-2 results in the activation and degranulation of mast cells, and LL-37 also activates immune cells, leading to inflammation and angiogenesis. Endoplasmic reticulum (ER) stress is induced by the trigger factors of rosacea. These factors include UV irradiation, barrier defects, and TRPs that are activated by heat, cold, irritants, acid, capsaicin, and resveratrol. ER stress increases the expression of LL-37. UV light causes the release of LL-37 and dsRNA from the damaged keratinocytes. LL37:dsRNA complex increases expression of vascular adhesion molecules, resulting in inflammation.

References: Woo YR, Lim JH, Cho DH, Park HJ. Alcoholic dermatitis: molecular mechanisms and management of a chronic cutaneous inflammatory condition. *Int J Mol Sci*. 2016;17(9).
Plewig G, Melnik B, Chen W. Plewig and Kligman's acne and rosacea. Plewig and Kligman's Acne and Alcoholic Dermatitis, 4th ed. Switzerland: Springer International Publishing; 2019, P511–514.
Shi X et al. Keratinocytes express cytokines and nerve growth factor in response to neuropeptide activation of the ERK1/2 and JNK MAPK transcription pathways. *Regul Pept*. 2013;186:92–103.

IL-17 induces angiogenesis.[23,24] Skin barrier defect is also involved in inflammation. *Demodex* can damage the epidermal barrier by biting on keratinocytes or through TLR-2 or KLK-5 (serine protease) induction.[27] Dysregulation of immune response leads to inflammation causing papulopustules and erythema (Figure 20).

Neurovascular dysregulation is induced by external stimuli such as cold, heat, exercise, stress, emotional changes, drinking alcohol, consuming spicy food, and chemicals that stimulate transient receptor potential channels (TRPs). Two nerve systems, afferent sensory nerve and skin sympathetic cholinergic nerve, are crucial in the pathogenesis of rosacea erythema, flushing, and neurogenic inflammation. Hairy skin contains sympathetic adrenergic and cholinergic fibers differently distributed around the skin. The sympathetic cholinergic fibers around the skin arterioles express acetylcholine, vasoactive intestinal peptide (VIP), pituitary adenylate-cyclase-activating polypeptide (PACAP), substance P, CGRP, and NO.[28–30] Activation of TRPs leads to the release of CGRP and substance P from afferent sensory neuron, triggering vasodilation and vascular permeability, activating mast cells, macrophages, and neutrophils, and resulting in subsequent neuroinflammatory responses.[23,29] TRPs can be found in nerve endings, keratinocytes, and endothelium. In the epidermis, cutaneous primary sensory afferents release substance P and CGRP. These neuropeptides bind and activate their cognate receptors on the keratinocyte and stimulate keratinocyte proliferation, substance P and CGRP expression, and secretion, respectively (Figure 21).[31] A study found that TRPV4 is a key driver for mast cell-mediated skin inflammation in *rosacea*. Mast cells significantly increase their expression of TRPV4 in response to LL37.[32]

In terms of triggering factors, the neurovascular responses in rosacea induced by anxiety, stress, heat, exercise, spicy food, and cold include the skin sympathetic cholinergic nerve, sensory nerve, and NO (Figure 22). Acute anxiety and stress activate sympathetic nervous system, causing cutaneous vasoconstriction and heat production through brown adipose tissue, leading to an increase in core body temperature.[33] During exercise, 80% of the energy generated by skeletal muscles is converted into heat, such as heat stimulation to the general body, and leads to a rise in the core body temperature.[28–30] Spicy food triggering gustatory reflex may affect the body via the same pathway. Spicy food can activate TRPV1 through the taste reflexes, and signals are sent to the primary gustatory center and the autonomic region of the insula. This exhibits finger tip temperature increase.[34] Meanwhile, experiments have confirmed that cheek vasodilation caused by spicy food is not associated with the parasympathetic nerve.[35] The rise in the core body temperature activates skin sympathetic cholinergic nerves to release vasoactive substances, leading to vasodilation in the hairy skin.[28–30] Prolonged exercise thermogenesis

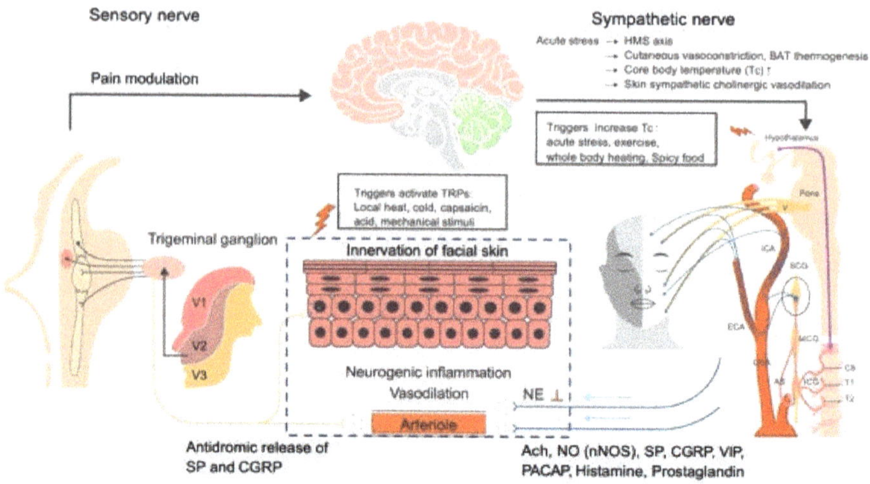


**Figure 21.** Innervation of skin sympathetic nerve and afferent sensory nerve. The superior cervical ganglion gives rise to the carotid plexus, whose fibers run with the carotid arteries and provide sympathetic innervation to the head. The free trigeminal nerve endings innervate the facial skin, including the epidermis and dermis. Acute stress activates the hypothalamic–medullary sympathetic (HMS) axis, causing cutaneous vasoconstriction and brown adipose tissue (BAT) thermogenesis, subsequently raising core body temperature (Tc). Increase in Tc activates skin sympathetic cholinergic nerve leading to cutaneous vasodilation and inhibition of sympathetic vasoconstriction. Exercise, whole-body heating, and spicy food also increase Tc. The mediators include, NO, SP, VIP, PACAP, histamine, and prostaglandin. The TRPs of afferent sensory nerves are activated by local heat, cold, capsaicin, acid, and mechanical stimuli causing antidromic release of SP and CGRP to the dermal arterioles and epidermis.

and local thermal stimulation within 42°C can activate TRPV1 in the sensory nerve and lead to antidromic release of CGRP and substance P, finally causing vasodilation.[29] Holzer et al. showed that NO may facilitate the release of CGRP from afferent nerve fibers or be a secondary vasorelaxant messenger of the peptide.[36]

As the temperature continues to rise, heat shock proteins are produced in blood vessels, subsequently causing the production of NO, which results in prolonged plateau vasodilation.[28–30] Local stimulation of capsaicin also activates TRPV1, and cold stimulation activates TRPA1, and both trigger the afferent sensory nerve response.[37] Although the aforementioned three vasodilations are normal physiological responses to dissipate heat, patients with rosacea have exacerbated reactions. Studies have

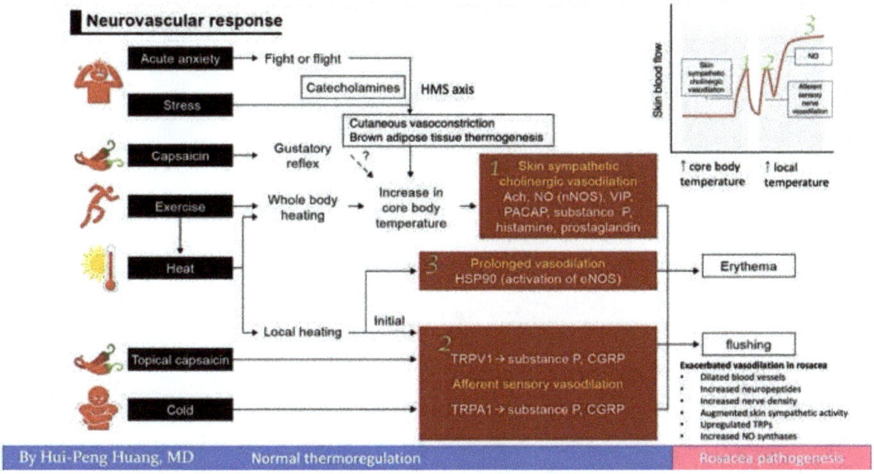


**Figure 22.** Enhancement of normal thermoregulation and neurovascular response in rosacea. Acute anxiety or stress activates the hypothalamic medullary-sympathetic (HMS) axis, causing cutaneous vasoconstriction and brown adipose tissue thermogenesis and then raising the core body temperature (Tc). Capsaicin, exercise, and whole-body heating also increases Tc. An increase in Tc leads to skin sympathetic cholinergic vasodilation.

Exercise also increases local temperature along with local heating causing biphasic vasodilation. The first peak is afferent sensory vasodilation, which is also activated by topical capsaicin and cold stimuli. When local heat continuously rises, a prolonged vasodilation with a plateau appears. Rosacea skin has predisposing factors that enhance the vasodilation to erythema and flushing.

showed that the skin sympathetic activity,[38] blood vessel dilation,[39] neuropeptides,[39] sensory nerve density in the dermis,[40] TRP expression,[41] and NO synthases are significantly increased in rosacea skin compared with those in normal skin (Figure 22).[42]

Overall, the pathophysiological pathways for rosacea are complicated. In summary, the pathways can be categorized into five components, having their triggers, receptors, and key mediators as: (1) prolonged vasodilation with nitric oxide; (2) afferent sensory vasodilation and neurological inflammation with TRPs, substance P, and CGRP; (3) immune-associated inflammation and vasodilation with TLR-2, endoplasmic reticulum (ER) stress, and LL37; (4) other non-neuronal inflammation and vasodilation and inflammation with vascular adhesion molecules; and (5) skin sympathetic cholinergic vasodilation with VIP and PACAP. As a mnemonic, we propose calling it the PAINS five subpathways of rosacea (Figure 23). The enhanced

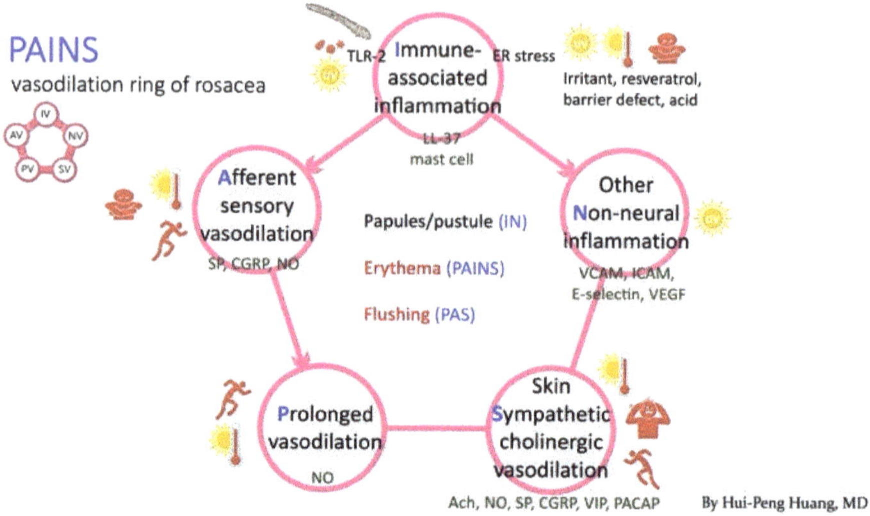


**Figure 23.** The "PAINS" vasodilation star of rosacea. The pathophysiological pathways for rosacea can be categorized into five components with their triggers. The involved receptors and key mediators are as follows: (1) Prolonged vasodilation with nitric oxide; (2) afferent sensory vasodilation and neurological inflammation with TRPs, substance P, and CGRP; (3) immune-associated inflammation and vasodilation with TLR-2, ER stress, and LL37; (4) Other non-neuronal inflammation and vasodilation and inflammation with vascular adhesion molecules; and (5) skin sympathetic cholinergic vasodilation with VIP and PACAP. All components cause erythema, but PAS also lead to flushing. PAINS: P, prolonged vasodilation; A, afferent sensory vasodilation; I, immune-associated vasodilation; N, other non-neuronal vasodilation; S, skin sympathetic cholinergic vasodilation.

sympathetic nerve, prolonged nerve (NO), and sensory nerve vasodilation responses lead to facial erythema and flushing in rosacea. In clinical application, performing arithmetic tasks to test sympathetic flushing, blowing air using hair dryer for afferent sensory flushing, and checking the history of flushing during prolonged exercise can be used to ensure a NO prolonged flushing.

Neurovascular dysregulation and immune response dysregulation are related to each other (crosstalk). Our published paper on the effective treatment of rosacea erythema with anti-*Demodex* medications indirectly proves this argument.[20] Increased expressions of VEGF in rosacea skin are also responsible for erythema and angiogenesis. The level of inducible nitric oxide synthase (iNOS) in the skin with ETR is higher than that of healthy skin.[42] Erythema alleviation has been found 30 minutes after intramuscular injection of nitric oxide (NO) scavenger, hydroxocobalamin, proving that NO is involved in erythema.[26]

In terms of microbes, the role of *Demodex* is the most predominant, and its discussion can be found in Section 1.3.2. Some studies also highlighted the roles of other microbes, such as *Staphylococcus epidermidis*,[43,44] *Bacillus oleronius*,[45] *Helicobacter pylori*,[46] and small intestinal bacteria.[47] The chitin in the exoskeleton of the *Demodex* can trigger innate immune responses, leading to an increase in the expression of TLR-2 and proinflammatory cytokines.[48]

In addition, in vitro studies have found that *Demodex* allergens can stimulate inflammasomes and contribute to the activation of the inflammatory cytokine IL-1β.[49] Some studies have also highlighted that proteins produced by *B. oleronius*, a bacterium associated with *Demodex*, can activate neutrophils.[50] *Bacillus oleronius* may also induce the differentiation of immune cells and promote the secretion of cathelicidin, MMP-9, TNF, IL-8, and other substances.[51]

Studies have found genetic predispositions to rosacea. Genes related to the rosacea in the studies include rs763035 intergenic between HLA-DRA and BTNL2; rs3733631 in TACR3; R702W in NOD2/CARD15; Glutathione S-transferase gene; polymorphisms of rs11168271 (Apal), rs731336 (TaqI), and rs11568820 (Cdx2) in the Vitamin D receptor; and polymorphisms in the VEGF gene.[24,52]

## Abbreviations

- CGRP: Calcitonin gene-related peptide
- CXCL: C-X-C motif chemokine ligand family
- hCAP 18: human cationic antimicrobial protein
- HSP 90: Heat shock protein 90
- KLK5: Kallikrein 5
- IL-6: Interleukin 6
- MMP 1: matrix metalloproteinase-1
- NO: Nitric oxide
- nNOS: Neuronal nitric oxide synthase

- PACAP: Pituitary adenylate-cyclase-activating polypeptide
- PAR 2: Protease-activated receptor 2
- ROS: Reactive oxygen species
- Th1: Type 1 T helper cells
- TLR-2: Toll-like receptor 2
- TNF: Tumor necrosis factor
- TRPs: Transient receptor potential families
- TRPV1: Transient Receptor Potential Vanilloid 1
- VEGF: vascular endothelial growth factor
- VIP: Vasoactive intestinal peptide

### 1.3.2 *Demodex as a trigger factor of rosacea and its control*

The DMD of a patient with rosacea is higher than that of control group,[14–17] and 82%–92% of patients with rosacea have a DMD higher than the diagnostic threshold.[16,18] According to the findings by Dr. Huang Hui-Peng, clinical features of demodicosis, such as papulopustules, white follicular plugs and scales or large pores, could be seen in some of these patients, whereas the other patients did not have any relevant clinical features.

In terms of treatment options, Sattler et al. in 2015 analyzed the therapeutic effect of topical metronidazole combined with systemic tetracyclines on rosacea and found that 72% of patients could achieve complete clinical clearance or a major reduction of papulopustules; however, DMD decreased only by 30%.[53] The result shows that combined treatment alleviates clinical symptoms but has limited effect on eradicating mites. In another study, the therapeutic effects of 5% permethrin and 0.75% metronidazole were compared and the results showed that they had similar erythema reduction scores. Regarding papule and pustule reduction, permethrin showed a slightly better effect than metronidazole, but there was no statistically significant difference between them. Regarding *Demodex* reduction, there is a significant difference between them, with topical permethrin reducing the *Demodex* level by up to 70%, but metronidazole only reducing it by 23%.[54]

Another study highlighted the difference in the efficacy of 1% ivermectin cream and 0.75% metronidazole cream. After 16 weeks of treatment, ivermectin showed better improvement in inflammatory lesions than metronidazole.[55] This study also found that as the treatment duration increased, the decrease in inflammatory lesions also increased significantly, which means that the effectiveness of treatment is closely related to time.[56] This study also followed the patients for 36 weeks and found that the patients receiving ivermectin had a median disease-free period of 3.8 months, which was longer than the group receiving metronidazole whose median was 2.8 months.[56] In addition to the effect of treatment duration on the efficacy, Schaller et al. showed that when the patient's DMD is higher than 100 mites/cm$^2$, patients with papules and pustules, treated with ivermectin, have better improvement than patients with a lower DMD.[57] Dr. Huang Hui-Peng found that in patients with mild and moderate ETR who also had a high DMD, ivermectin 1% cream effectively improved erythema on the face; moreover, the reduction in Clinician's Erythema Assessment (CEA) grade and the reduction in the DMD were positively correlated (Spearman's rho = 0.501, p = 0.002, n = 36).[20] In terms of the efficacy of oral ivermectin, studies have found that combined treatment with metronidazole is more effective than ivermectin alone. After 4 weeks of treatment, DMD in the group receiving single medicine only dropped by 40%; in the combined medicine group, DMD could drop as high as 90%.[58] Regarding treatment with other drugs, benzyl benzoate is more irritating and requires a longer treatment duration to achieve the curative effect;[59] thus, it is used less frequently.

Based on data not yet published, in Taiwan, Dr. Huang Hui-Peng recruited a total of 453 patients with rosacea and high DMD from January to December 2018 to study the outcomes of topical ivermectin alone or in combination with other treatments, with a follow-up period to March 2022. Except for patients who received their treatment longer than 5 months, dropped off during follow-up, and had no recurrence, 63 of the remaining 107 patients were selected for further study. These 63 patients had complete recordings of their DMD at the beginning and end of their treatment, as well as at the time of recurrence.

The study findings showed that the average interval between two treatments in the study population was 21.6 months, and the average DMD dropped from 172.5 to 8.1 mites/cm$^2$ after treatment. The average papulopustular-free time (disease-free time) was 17 months, and the median was about 14 months. The DMD at the time of recurrence was

95.6 mites/cm$^2$, which was lower than the original density before treatment. The time from symptom recurrence to medical treatment ranged from 1 day to 3 weeks. It is speculated that after patients have their first treatment, when they feel uncomfortable during relapse, they visit a doctor immediately; thus, their DMD has not increased to a very high level. Another analysis by Dr. Huang Hui-Peng involving 35 patients with PPR receiving topical ivermectin alone or in combination with other treatments showed that there was no significant difference in the total amount of ivermectin 1% cream between the successful treatment group and the improvement group. Nevertheless, the average treatment duration was significantly different, where the average treatment durations were 8.0 ± 3.8 weeks and 4.8 ± 1.9 weeks, respectively. This result showed that the longer the treatment duration, the higher the chance of curing papulopustules. In addition, the DMD after treatment was also relatively low, 7.5 ± 2.2/cm$^2$ in the successful treatment group and 23.4 ± 10.7 cm$^2$ in the improvement group, showing that if a lower DMD can be achieved after treatment, a better outcome can be expected.

Based on the above findings summarized in Table 3, we found that, after treatment for rosacea begins, the number of papulopustules is decreased together with the decreased DMD, and the average decrease proportion curves of the papulopustules and DMD are quite consistent.

The higher the decrease in the DMD, the higher the reduction in the number of papulopustules (Figure 24). The median duration of disease remission after rosacea treatment was 3.8 months with ivermectin cream compared with 2.8 months with metronidazole cream.[56] Synergistic treatment with ivermectin cream reduced the final DMD to normal values, with a median duration of 14 months, which was better than 3.8 months achieved by ivermectin alone without the DMD measured (Figure 25).

In conclusion, *Demodex* is an important trigger factor for rosacea and should be considered in its clinical control. Because the prevalence rate of *Demodex* in patients with ETR and PPR is as high as 82%–92% clinically, patients who may have high DMD can be targeted based on their symptoms and subtypes of rosacea, and further tests can be conducted to confirm such cases. Topical ivermectin is recommended when patients have high DMD, either alone or in combination with other symptomatic treatments.

**Table 3.** Summary of treatment effect of rosacea

| Treatment | Case No. | Treatment duration | Papules/ pustules | Erythema | Demodex density | Median time to first relapse | Authors |
|---|---|---|---|---|---|---|---|
| Topical MTN gel + tetracyclines | 25 | 53.5 days (21–112) | 72% success | NA | –30% | NA | Turgut et al.[18] |
| Permethrin 5% | 20 | 60 days | –71%/–76% | CEA 2.60 →1.34 | –70% | NA | Koçak et al.[54] |
| Topical MTN gel 0.75% | 20 | | –64%/–51% | CEA 2.85 →1.40 | –23% | | Koçak et al.[54] |
| Topical ivermectin 1% | 478 | 16 weeks | –83% | NA | NA | 3.8 months | Taieb et al.[55,56] |
| Topical MTN cream 0.75% | 484 | | –73.7% | NA | NA | 2.8 months | Taieb et al.[55,56] |
| Topical ivermectin 1%‡ | 20 | 12 weeks | –82% | NA | –99% | NA | Schaller et al.[57] |
| Topical ivermectin 1% + carvedilol‡ | 12 | 1–12 weeks | NA | CEA 1.9 → 1.1 ER 64 | –66% | NA | Huang et al.[20] |
| Combined treatments‡ | 63 | 2–20 weeks | NA | NA | –95% | 14 months* | Hui-Peng Huang (unpublished) |
| Oral ivermectin | 15 | 2 doses/2 weeks | 78.3% success† | NA | –40% | NA | Salem et al.[58] |
| Oral ivermectin + metronidazole | 15 | Evaluate at 4th week | 98.3% success† | NA | –90% | NA | Salem et al.[58] |

ER, Excellent response; MTN, metronidazole; Success, complete clear and almost clear (major or marked improvement); *Patients with a final mean *Demodex* density 8.1 mites/$cm^2$ by the thumbnail-squeezing method; †, Acne, rosacea, POD, and blepharitis altogether; ‡, High *Demodex* density.

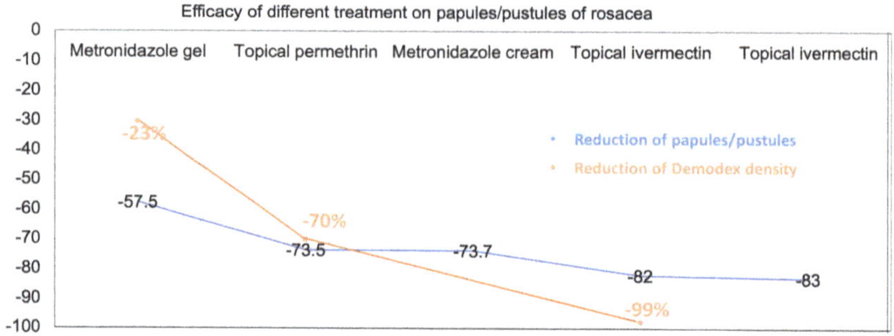


| | Metronidazole gel 0.75% | Topical permethrin 5% | Metronidazole cream 0.75% | Topical ivermectin 1% | Topical ivermectin 1% |
|---|---|---|---|---|---|
| Treatment duration | 60 days (8.6 weeks) | 60 days (8.6 weeks) | 16 weeks | 12 weeks | 16 weeks |
| Authors | Turgut et al.[18] (2015) | Koçak et al.[54] 2002 | Taieb et al.[55,56] (2015) | Schaller et al.[57] (2017) | Taieb et al.[55,56] (2015) |

**Figure 24.** After rosacea treatment, the number of papulopustules was decreased together with the decreased *Demodex* density.

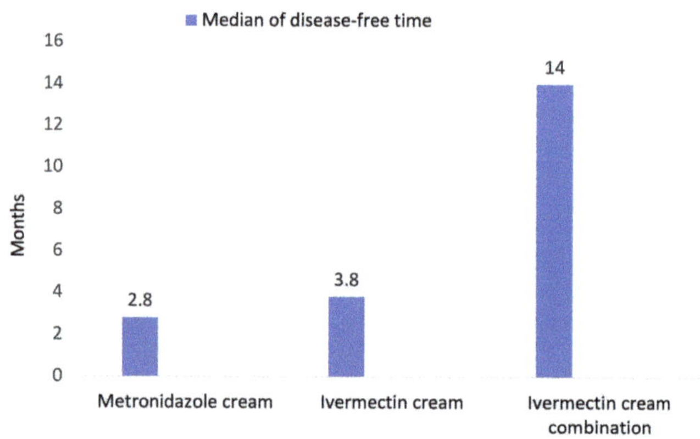


| Treatment duration | 16 weeks | 16 weeks | 2-20 weeks |
|---|---|---|---|
| Demodex | Not available | Not available | 172→ 8/cm$^2$ |
| Authors | Taieb et al. (2015)[55,56] | Taieb et al. (2015)[55,56] | Hui-Peng Huang unpublished |

**Figure 25.** Comparison of the median duration of disease remission after rosacea treatment showed that ivermectin cream efficacy was superior to that of metronidazole cream. Combination treatment with ivermectin cream reduced the final *Demodex* density to normal values, with a median symptom-free time of 14 months, which was better than 3.8 months achieved by ivermectin alone without the *Demodex* density measured.

### 1.3.3 *Introduction to Demodex*

*Demodex* is an ectoparasite with four pairs of legs. Its transmission is species-specific, i.e., human *Demodex* is not transmitted to other animals across species, and *Demodex* of cats and dogs is not transmitted to humans. Human *Demodex* species include *Demodex folliculorum* and *Demodex brevis. Demodex folliculorum* lives in the shallowest layer of hair follicles, called infundibulum. At this location, it makes a living by biting the keratinocytes and sebum of hair follicles (Figures 26 and 27). *Demodex brevis* feeds on sebum and infests in sebaceous glands, particularly the sebaceous duct. The meibomian glands of the eyelids are also sites where *D. brevis* is parasitic. Some studies distinguish them based on their body sizes, while others distinguish them based on their body transparency. Doctor Zhou from Xi'an Jiaotong University analyzed the mitochondrial 16 SrDNA of *Demodex* and found that the shape of the tail is the most reliable morphology for differentiation. *Demodex folliculorum* has a blunt tail like a finger, and *D. brevis* has a sharp tail like a cone. Some *D. folliculorum* individuals are smaller than *D. brevis*.[60] The

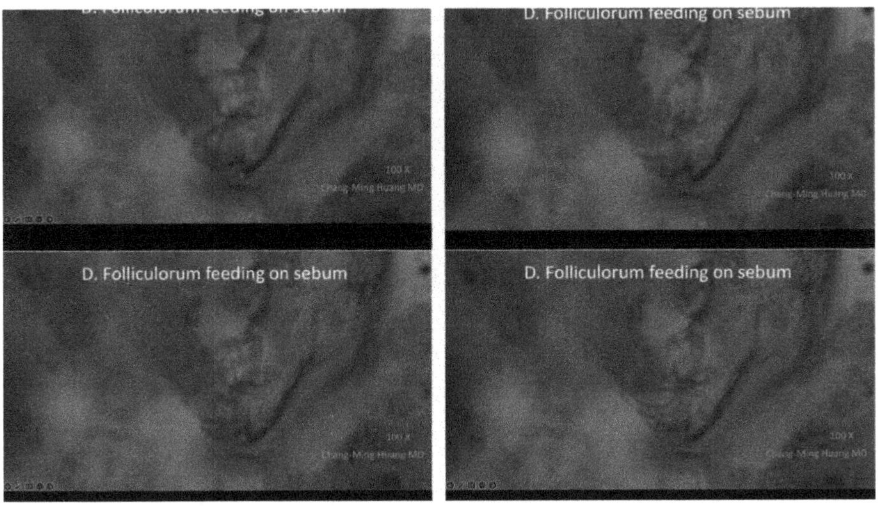


**Figure 26.** A time-lapse photograph shows *D. folliculorum* feeding on sebum. The image was obtained by collecting a tissue sample using the thumbnail-squeezing method. YouTube link: *Demodex folliculorum* feeds on sebum. https://youtu.be/KdMDGT9BMbQ?si=gjmW23eOuzAAvYLv

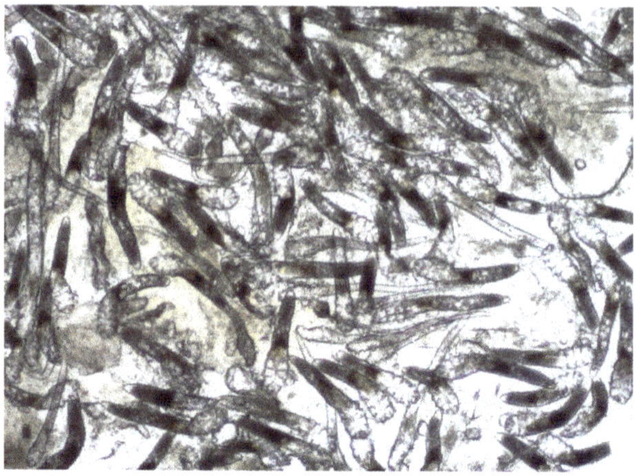

**Figure 27.** Densely packed *Demodex* mites obtained from the face by the thumbnail-squeezing method.

parasitic location of *Demodex* is mainly on the face, particularly the cheeks, nose, glabella, and chin, where sebaceous glands are highly distributed. A small number of *Demodex* mites can also be sampled from the scalp, body, and neck because *Demodex* mites live in hair follicles and sebaceous glands and are considered external parasites. The average size of adult *D. folliculorum* is twice that of *D. brevis*. The body length of *D. folliculorum* is 0.3–0.4 mm, whereas the body length of *D. brevis* is 0.15–0.2 mm. A small number of *Demodex* mites are not considered to harm human bodies; however, when their number exceeds a certain level, they may cause skin damage, which is called demodicosis. Demodicosis can be differentiated into primary and secondary demodicosis, where the latter is accompanied by general or local immunosuppression.[19]

The main cause of *Demodex* proliferation is immune suppression, such as using steroids or innate immune dysfunction. Some online articles also mention oil-containing skin care products and epidermal damage as causes. From my personal view, more evidence is needed to support these arguments. The routes of transmission are via skin, hair, and eyelash contact. *Demodex* in newborns comes from close contact with the parents' facial skin. According to our experimental observations, *Demodex* dies in a few hours to a day in a dry environment. However, they can survive for 4–5 days in a very humid environment. Therefore, there is less concern about quilts and pillows. However, sharing damp towels may be a route of transmission. Fortunately, people with normal immunity are not particularly susceptible to *Demodex* and can keep their numbers under control. The chance of parents and children having excessive levels of *Demodex* is higher than the chance of a couple having high levels of *Demodex*. A possible explanation is that parents and children have similar innate immune responses. The prevalence of *Demodex* in normal people varies depending on age groups. The paper, "Thumbnail-squeezing method: an effective method for assessing *Demodex* density in rosacea," co-authored by Dr. Huang Hui-Peng, Prof. Hsu Chao-Kai, and Prof. Lee Yu-Yun, shows that 69.3% of healthy people aged 16–68 years could be found with *Demodex*, compared with the percentage at 99%–100% in patients with rosacea. The normal value is <12 mites/cm$^2$.[16]

On June 24, 2022, the Chinese version of BBC News published a report on human *Demodex* and provided some popular scientific knowledge about *Demodex*. However, its content deviated in some places from *Demodex* known to dermatologists. The report claimed that *Demodex* is a skin cleaner. The comments included that humans should be willing to provide a home for *D. folliculorum* and establish a close relationship with them; they are tiny and cute; there should be no concern about them; they clean our pores and keep them smooth; and they do no harm to humans.

As shown by the biopsy, *Demodex* mites eat the keratinocytes of hair follicles.[27] In our experiments, we observed and photographed *Demodex* mites biting the sebum (Figure 26). It is not clear whether *Demodex* mites eat keratin or not. The mere discovery of *Demodex* feeding on live keratinocytes is sufficient to negate the claims of harmless nature of *Demodex*.

"As their genetic diversity decreases, their dependence on us increases; which means that they may be at risk of extinction." The fact is that *Demodex* cannot infest across species. This dependence does not affect its survival. As long as there are humans, they do not face the risk of extinction. "Our long-standing relationship with *Demodex* has led them to develop aspects that are beneficial to humans, such as keeping our pores from getting clogged." This statement is not supported by research. There are numerous clinical cases whose pores were blocked by *Demodex* mites (Figures 11, 12) and could only be unblocked after antiparasitic treatments.

Using the TSM we proposed, it is not rare to find cases with >500 *Demodex* mites/cm$^2$ of their skin, which was damaged, far from smooth or healthy. There are 250–270 hair follicles/cm$^2$ of skin on the human face. *Demodex* mites do not follow a normal distribution but are unevenly clustered in the hair follicles. The cheeks, nose, chin, and forehead (glabella) are the areas with the highest DMD. A small number of *Demodex* mites are tolerable to the skin and considered harmless, which we can coexist with.

For an excessive number of *Demodex* mites that alter the skin, immediate intervention is required. Skin features include papules, pustules, large pores, and fine white plugs in the pores. There can also be various combinations and varying degrees of the above features. When patients see the densely packed *Demodex* mites on their faces (Figure 27), they are often shocked and find it unbelievable that some say *Demodex* is harmless. The article also mentioned that D. folliculorum does not do much harm to the human body; on the contrary, it helps clean pores and keeps our skin smooth. Adding the words "a small number" to this sentence makes it a factual statement. The lack of these few words makes a huge difference!

### 1.3.4 *Rosacea treatment: something as important as Demodex*

According to the NRS in the US, the main factors contributing to the exacerbation of rosacea are as follows: ultraviolet (UV) rays 81%, emotional factors 79%, heat 75%, strong winds 57%, strenuous exercise 56%, alcohol 52%, hot baths 51%, cold weather 46%, spicy foods 45%, and humidity 44%. Other factors include hot and stuffy indoors 41%, improper skin care products 41%, hot drinks 36%, cosmetics 27%, medicines 15%, citrus fruits 13%, pickled meats 10%, and dairy products 8% (https://www.rosacea.org/patients/rosacea-triggers/rosacea-triggers-survey).

UV rays, emotional factors, and heat are major factors. Our findings show that 92% of patients with rosacea were found with *Demodex*. Thus, in addition to *Demodex*, other factors must also be dealt with together to complete the treatment (Figure 28). Diet accounts for a relatively minor factor. Diet intervention should only be involved when there are clear signs of deterioration so that the impact on the quality of life can be controlled.

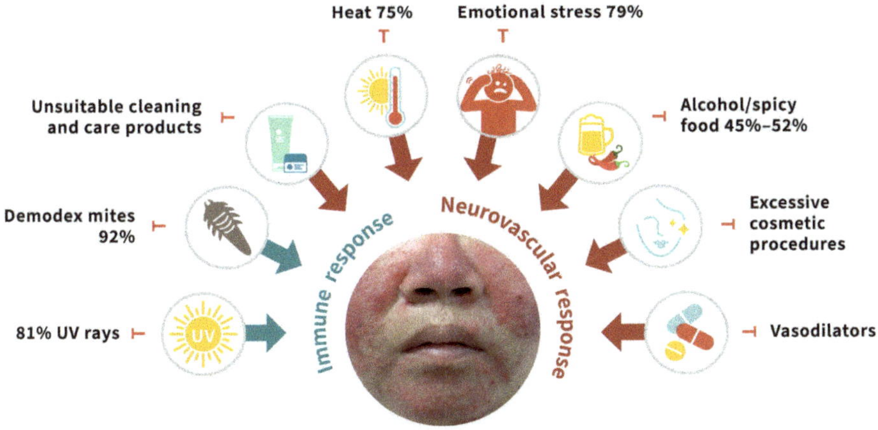


**Figure 28.** Rosacea treatment — something as important as *Demodex*. Ultraviolet (UV) rays and *Demodex* induce immune responses. Heat stimulation, emotional stress, alcohol, spicy food, and vasodilators cause neurovascular responses. Excessive cosmetic procedures and inappropriate cleansing and skin care products destroy the epidermal barrier and cause facial erythema.

## References

1. Crawford GH, Pelle MT, James WD. Rosacea: I. Etiology, pathogenesis, and subtype classification. *J Am Acad Dermatol.* 2004;51(3):327–341.
2. Heisig M, Reich A. Psychosocial aspects of rosacea with a focus on anxiety and depression. *Clin Cosmet Investig Dermatol.* 2018;11:103–107.
3. Dai R, Lin B, Zhang X, Lou Y, Xu S. Depression and anxiety in alcoholic dermatitis patients: A systematic review and meta-analysis. *Dermatol Ther.* 2021;11(6):2089–2105.
4. Marson JW, Baldwin HE. Rosacea: A wholistic review and update from pathogenesis to diagnosis and therapy. *Int J Dermatol.* 2020;59(6):e175–e182.
5. Tan J, Schöfer H, Araviiskaia E, Audibert F, Kerrouche N, Berg M. Prevalence of rosacea in the general population of Germany and Russia- The RISE study. *J Eur Acad Dermatol Venereol.* 2016;30(3):428–434.
6. Tan J, Almeida LM, Bewley A, et al. Updating the diagnosis, classification and assessment of rosacea: Recommendations from the global ROSacea COnsensus (ROSCO) panel. *Br J Dermatol.* 2017;176(2):431–438.
7. Gallo RL, Granstein RD, Kang S, et al. Standard classification and pathophysiology of rosacea: The 2017 update by the National Alcoholic Dermatitis Society Expert Committee. *J Am Acad Dermatol.* 2018;78(1):148–155.

8. Schaller M, Almeida LMC, Bewley A, et al. Recommendations for rosacea diagnosis, classification and management: Update from the global ROSacea COnsensus 2019 panel. *Br J Dermatol.* 2020;182(5):1269–1276.
9. Kim HO, Kang SY, Kim KE, Cho SY, Kim KH, Kim IH. Neurogenic rosacea in Korea. *J Dermatol.* 2021;48(1):49–55.
10. Sadeghian A, Rouhana H, Oswald-Stumpf B, Boh E. Etiologies and management of cutaneous flushing: Nonmalignant causes. *J Am Acad Dermatol.* 2017;77(3):391–402.
11. Brown R, Macefield VG. Skin sympathetic nerve activity in humans during exposure to emotionally-charged images: sex differences. *Front Physiol.* 2014;5:111.
12. Sadeghian A, Rouhana H, Oswald-Stumpf B, Boh E. Etiologies and management of cutaneous flushing: Malignant causes. *J Am Acad Dermatol.* 2017;77(3):405–414.
13. Odo ME, Odo LM, Farias RV, et al. Botulinum toxin for the treatment of menopausal hot flushes: A pilot study. *Dermatol Surg.* 2011;37(11):1579–1583.
14. Forton F, Seys B. Density of *Demodex folliculorum* in rosacea: A case-control study using standardized skin-surface biopsy. *Br J Dermatol.* 1993;128(6):650–659.
15. Forton FM, De Maertelaer V. Two consecutive standardized skin surface biopsies: An improved sampling method to evaluate *Demodex* density as a diagnostic tool for alcoholic dermatitis and demodicosis. *Acta Derm Venereol.* 2017;97(2):242–248.
16. Huang HP, Hsu CK, Lee JY. Thumbnail-squeezing method: An effective method for assessing *Demodex* density in rosacea. *J Eur Acad Dermatol Venereol.* 2020;34(7):e343–e345.
17. Huang HP, Hsu CK, Lee JY. A new superficial needle-scraping method for assessing *Demodex* density in papulopustular rosacea. *J Cosmet Dermatol.* 2020;19(4):896–900.
18. Turgut Erdemir A, Gurel MS, Koku Aksu AE, Falay T, Inan Yuksel E, Sarikaya E. *Demodex* mites in acne rosacea: Reflectance confocal microscopic study. *Australas J Dermatol.* 2017;58(2):e26–e30.
19. Chen W, Plewig G. Human demodicosis: Revisit and a proposed classification. *Br J Dermatol.* 2014;17(6):1219–1225.
20. Huang HP, Hsu CK, Lee JY. Rosacea with persistent facial erythema and high *Demodex* density effectively treated with topical ivermectin alone or combined with oral carvedilol. *Dermatol Ther.* 2021;34(2):e14899.

21. Huang HP, Hsu CK, Lee JY. Topical ivermectin-induced transient flare of rosacea as a host reaction to killed *Demodex* mites preventable by short-term use of topical corticosteroid. *Dermatologic therapy.* 2022;35(7):e15517.
22. Qudsiya Z, Waseem M. Dermatomyositis. [Updated 2023 Aug 7]. In: StatPearls [Internet]. Treasure Island (FL): StatPearls Publishing; 2024 Jan-. Available from: https://www.ncbi.nlm.nih.gov/books/NBK558917/
23. Rodrigues-Braz D, Zhao M, Yesilirmak N, Aractingi S, Behar-Cohen F, Bourges JL. Cutaneous and ocular rosacea: Common and specific physiopathogenic mechanisms and study models. *Mol Vis.* 2021;27:323–353.
24. Woo YR, Lim JH, Cho DH, Park HJ. Rosacea: Molecular mechanisms and management of a chronic cutaneous inflammatory condition. *Int J Mol Sci.* 2016;17(9).
25. Moura AKA, Guedes F, Rivitti-Machado MC, Sotto MN. Innate immunity in rosacea. Langerhans cells, plasmacytoid dendritic cells, Toll-like receptors and inducible oxide nitric synthase (iNOS) expression in skin specimens: case-control study. *Arch Dermatol Res.* 2018;310(2):139–146.
26. Huang YW, Huang HP, Hsu CK, Lee JY. Hydroxocobalamin: An effective treatment for flushing and persistent erythema in rosacea. *J Clin Aesthet Dermatol.* 2022;15(6):42–45.
27. Forton FM. Papulopustular rosacea, skin immunity and *Demodex*: pityriasis folliculorum as a missing link. *J Eur Acad Dermatol Venereol.* 2012; 26: 19–28.
28. Kellogg DL, Jr., Pérgola PE, Piest KL, et al. Cutaneous active vasodilation in humans is mediated by cholinergic nerve cotransmission. *Circ Res.* 1995;77(6):1222–1228.
29. Kellogg DL, Jr. In vivo mechanisms of cutaneous vasodilation and vasoconstriction in humans during thermoregulatory challenges. *J Appl Physiol.* 2006;100(5):1709–1718.
30. Yamazaki F, Minokoshi K. Exercise training and cutaneous vasodilator function. *Jpn J Phys Fit Sports Med.* 2017;66:185–193.
31. Shi X, Wang L, Clark JD, Kingery WS. Keratinocytes express cytokines and nerve growth factor in response to neuropeptide activation of the ERK1/2 and JNK MAPK transcription pathways. *Regul Pept.* 2013;186:92–103.
32. Mascarenhas NL, Wang Z, Chang YL, Di Nardo A. TRPV4 Mediates. Mast Cell Activation in Cathelicidin-Induced Rosacea Inflammation. *J Invest Dermatol.* 2017;137:972–5.

33. Oka T. Psychogenic fever: how psychological stress affects body. temperature in the clinical population. *Temperature*. 2015;2:368–378.
34. Kawakami S, Sato H, Sasaki AT, et al. The brain mechanisms underlying the perception of pungent taste of capsaicin and the subsequent autonomic responses. *Front Hum Neurosci.* 2015;9:720.
35. Drummond PD. Mechanisms of physiological gustatory sweating and flushing in the face. *J Auton Nerv Syst.* 1995;52(2–3):117–124.
36. Holzer P, Wachter C, Heinemann A, Jocic M, Lippe IT, Herbert MK. Sensory nerves, nitric oxide and NANC vasodilatation. *Arch Int Pharmacodyn Ther.* 1995;329:67–79.
37. Aubdool AA, Brain SD. Neurovascular aspects of skin neurogenic. inflammation. *J Investig Dermatol Symp Proc.* 2011;15:33–39.
38. Metzler-Wilson K, Toma K, Sammons DL, Mann S, Jurovcik AJ, Demidova O, Wilson TE. Augmented supraorbital skin sympathetic nerve activity responses to symptom trigger events in rosacea patients. *J Neurophysiol.* 2015;114: 1530–1537.
39. Schwab VD, Sulk M, Seeliger S, Nowak P, Aubert J, Mess C, et al. Neurovascular and neuroimmune aspects in the pathophysiology of rosacea. *J Investig Dermatol Symp Proc.* 2011;15:53–62.
40. Rainer BM, Kang S, Chien AL. Rosacea: Epidemiology, pathogenesis, and treatment. *Dermatoendocrinol.* 2017;9:e1361574.
41. KTM Chen. Transient receptors potential (TRP) channels and. neuroimmunology Mutation pathways of Rosacea. *J Cell Sci Mutat.* 2018;2(1):39–42.
42. Moura AKA, Guedes F, Rivitti-Machado MC, Sotto MN. Inate immunity. in rosacea. Langerhans cells, plasmacytoid dentritic cells, Toll-like receptors and inducible oxide nitric synthase (iNOS) expression in skin specimens: case-control study. *Arch Dermatol Res.* 2018;310:139–146.
43. Whitfeld M, Gunasingam N, Leow LJ, Shirato K, Preda V. Staphylococcus epidermidis: a possible role in the pustules of rosacea. *J Am Acad Dermatol.* 2011;64(1):49–52.
44. Woo YR, Lee SH, Cho SH, Lee JD, Kim HS. Characterization and analysis of the skin microbiota in rosacea: impact of systemic antibiotics. *J Clin Med.* 2020;9.
45. Lacey N, Delaney S, Kavanagh K, Powell FC. Mite-related bacterial antigens stimulate inflammatory cells in rosacea. *Br J Dermatol.* 2007;157(3): 474–481.

46. Tüzün Y, Keskin S, Kote E. The role of Helicobacter pylori infection in skin diseases: facts and controversies. *Clin Dermatol.* 2010;28(5):478–482.
47. Drago F, Ciccarese G, Herzum A, Drago F, Rebora A, Parodi A. The association between cigarettes smoke, small intestine bacterial overgrowth and rosacea. *G Ital Dermatol Venereol.* 2019;154(6):727–728.
48. Roh KB, Ryu DH, Cho E, Weon JB, Park D, Kweon DH, Jung E. Coptis chinensis franch directly inhibits proteolytic activation of kallikrein 5 and cathelicidin associated with rosacea in epidermal keratinocytes. *Molecules.* 2020;25.
49. Chen C, Wang P, Zhang L, Liu X, Zhang H, Cao Y, Wang X, Zeng Q. Exploring the pathogenesis and mechanism-targeted treatments of rosacea: previous understanding and updates. *Biomedicines.* 2023;11.
50. McMahon F, Banville N, Bergin DA, Smedman C, Paulie S, Reeves E, Kavanagh K. Activation of neutrophils via IP3 pathway following exposure to *Demodex*-associated bacterial proteins. *Inflammation.* 2016;39:425–433.
51. Kim HS. Microbiota in rosacea. *Am J Clin Dermatol.* 2020;21:25–35.
52. Abram K, Silm H, Maaroos HI, Oona M. Risk factors associated with rosacea. *J Eur Acad Dermatol Venereol.* 2010;24(5):565–571.
53. Sattler EC, Hoffmann VS, Ruzicka T, Braunmühl TV, Berking C. Reflectance confocal microscopy for monitoring the density of *Demodex* mites in rosacea patients before and after treatment. *Br J Dermatol.* 2015;173(1):69–75.
54. Koçak M, Yali S, Vahapo lu G, Ekiolu M. Permethrin 5% cream versus metronidazole 0.75% gel for the treatment of papulopustular rosacea. A randomized double-blind placebo-controlled study. *Dermatology.* 2002;205(3):265–270.
55. Taieb A, Ortonne JP, Ruzicka T, et al. Superiority of ivermectin 1% cream over metronidazole 0.75% cream in treating inflammatory lesions of rosacea: a randomized, investigator-blinded trial. *Br J Dermatol.* 2015;172(4):1103–1110.
56. Taieb A, Khemis A, Ruzicka T, et al. Maintenance of remission following successful treatment of papulopustular rosacea with ivermectin 1% cream vs. metronidazole 0.75% cream: 36-week extension of the ATTRACT randomized study. *J Eur Acad Dermatol Venereol.* 2016;30(5):829–836.
57. Schaller M, Gonser L, Belge K, et al. Dual anti-inflammatory and anti-parasitic action of topical ivermectin 1% in papulopustular rosacea. *J Eur Acad Dermatol Venereol.* 2017;31(11):1907–1911.

58. Salem DA, El-Shazly A, Nabih N, El-Bayoumy Y, Saleh S. Evaluation of the efficacy of oral ivermectin in comparison with ivermectin-metronidazole combined therapy in the treatment of ocular and skin lesions of *Demodex folliculorum*. *Int J Infect Dis*. 2013;17(5):e343–347.
59. Forton FMN, De Maertelaer V. Treatment of rosacea and demodicosis with benzyl benzoate: effects of different doses on *Demodex* density and clinical symptoms. *J Eur Acad Dermatol Venereol*. 2020;34(2):365–369.
60. Zhao YE, Hu L, Ma JX. Molecular identification of four phenotypes of human *Demodex* mites (Acari: Demodicidae) based on mitochondrial 16S rDNA. *Parasitol Res*. 2013;112(11):3703–3711.

# 2

# My Journey into *Demodex* and Rosacea Research

## 2.1 Enlightenment

Before 2012, I had treated quite a few patients who suffered from recurring papulopustules on their faces. I had never felt that I was familiar with this disease until I saw a young lady who showed some scattered papulopustules on her face. This patient had been seeking treatments for 3 years, received negative results on skin patch tests, was treated with indomethacin for Ofuji's disease, and took metronidazole gel for rosacea. None of these interventions made an improvement. Later, I referred this patient to Prof. Lee Yu-Yun at the National Cheng Kung University Hospital. After scraping the pustules from the skin for a KOH test, Lee found a *Demodex* mite under the microscope and considered *Demodex* infestation. When her family members told me that *Demodex* was found, I was very interested and wanted to look them for myself. Thus, I picked up a blunt scalpel and scraped the pustules and found that the pustule fluid dried quickly on the scalpel, leaving me no tissue sample that I could transfer to a slide for examination. Subsequently, I came up with the idea of using an 18-gauge needle for taking a sample, to get enough pustule fluid for a microscopic observation. We performed the experiment and found that the patient was infested with *Demodex*. After treatment, she recovered and had never seen a relapse for a follow-up period of 8 years. After the experience with this patient, we found that there were many similar patients in the OPD clinic; thus, we gradually developed a method of using an 18-gauge needle to scrape pustules to examine *Demodex*.

## 2.2 The time before ivermectin cream treatment in Taiwan

As more and more patients with excessive *Demodex* mites were detected, the demand for treatment was increasing. Before 2016, limited drugs were available in Taiwan to treat *Demodex*, such as metronidazole gel 0.75%, crotamiton lotion 10%, crotamiton 10% + hydrocortisone 0.25% cream, benzyl benzoate lotion 20% (BBL), and r-BHC cream 1%. Among them, BBL has the most stable antiparasitic effect. Unfortunately, its application on the face causes pain, and the pain may even last for 20 minutes. BBL also has a strong smell of insecticide. During the treatment, the face becomes reddish and may form scales. One of my patients with rosacea, who was very cooperative, once returned to me and cried while talking, "Dr. Huang, I cannot stand it anymore. This insecticide lotion hurts when I apply it on my cheeks, and the whole house smells of insecticide." (Stories of Patients with Rosacea 1). Since that day, we tried many kinds of moisturizing products, including applying them before the BBL lotion, diluting the lotion and applying it, and applying it after the lotion, but nothing could reduce the pain and irritating smell. Later, we finally found that applying 50% tea tree oil after BBL application can eliminate the pain and smell, and the scaling problem can be improved by using a moisturizing cream. After 2–4 months of continuous treatment, no mites could be found in the test for another three consecutive weeks. The patients' skin became very smooth, delicate, and bright. Patients who completed the treatment were highly satisfied (Figure 29). Further follow-up revealed that many of them had sustained remission for more than 3 years and did not require any treatment. In the past, it was only possible to convince patients to accept this kind of antiparasitic drugs under two situations: (1) the patient has been using other treatment methods for a long time, which are ineffective or making the condition worse; (2) we need to use a lot of data and pictures to explain patients why the treatment is needed and what is expected, alongside some photos of patients showing skin improvement to smooth, to convince them that this treatment can be considered. This kind of health education usually takes 30 minutes (Figure 30).

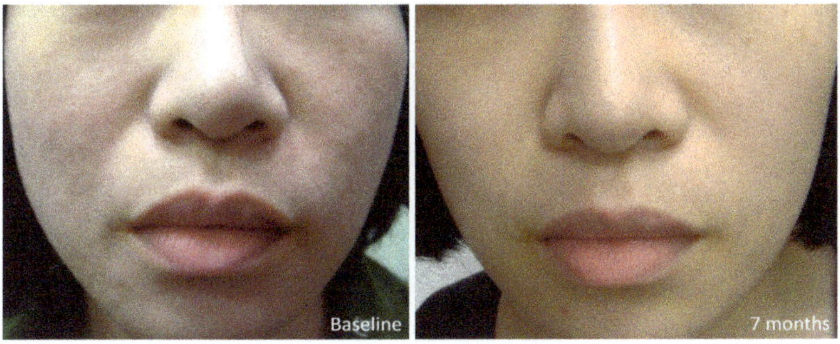


**Figure 29.** Rosacea before and after treatment. The patient's skin became very smooth, delicate, and bright.

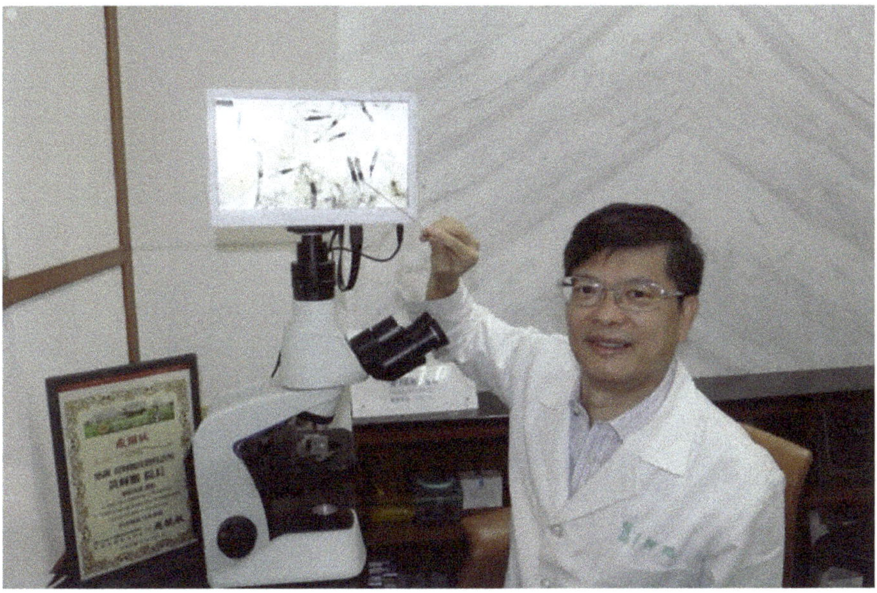

**Figure 30.** Patiently explaining the treatment to patients with images is the key to their acceptance of antiparasitic treatment.

We believe the time spent is worth it and are willing to do it because we have seen too many cases suffering from ineffective treatments or deterioration.

## 2.3 My patients and I on my *Demodex* journey (2012–2017)

Before 2017, the use of antiparasitic drugs during rosacea treatment was the only one of its kind in Taiwan (Figure 31). Therefore, patients with rosacea who had encountered difficulties with other treatments came from all over Taiwan, from the south to the north and even the east and outlying islands. After searching on the Internet, they came to Dr. Huang Hui-Peng Dermatology Clinic in Tainan city to seek medical help. There was a woman who had suffered from PPR for a long time. She was treated with traditional methods in my OPD clinic from 2012 to 2014, seeing no improvement but only exacerbation. One day, she called the clinic and asked us to wait for her because she wanted to be the last one to see the doctor. At 12 noon, she entered the consultation room and spoke to me very tearfully and in distress, "My face is like this. When my colleagues and friends see me, they ask me what is wrong and why I do not see a doctor. I know they care about me, but their words upset me. I follow suit and purchase whatever skincare products they recommend to me. However, none of the products work for me. What should I do?" We felt deep sympathy for her upon hearing her statements. Examinations showed that her rosacea was related to excessive *Demodex* mites. After our careful explanation to her, she started the treatment combining BBL, tea tree oil, and oral antibiotics. One month later, the papulopustules on her face had improved by more than 60%. Nine months later, we found through photo tracking that her facial skin had become smooth, delicate, and clear from papulopustules (Figure 32). She revisited the clinic three years later with very few signs of papulopustules, which were enough to increase her awareness for medical help. In addition, by the year 2017, a new antiparasitic drug has become available, enabling patients to see substantial improvement after two months of easy-to-apply treatment. Patients no longer needed to undergo intensive treatment as they did in the past.

Before 2017, there were some medical reports on using antiparasitic drugs to kill *Demodex* mites to treat rosacea, but this practice was not a mainstream treatment. Therefore, we faced resistance and criticism, as you can imagine. Some patients had finally received our suggestion of anti-*Demodex* treatment this time but came back to question us the next time after visiting other doctors or pharmacists who criticized our treatment by saying things like "how is it possible to use this drug on the face," "*Demodex*

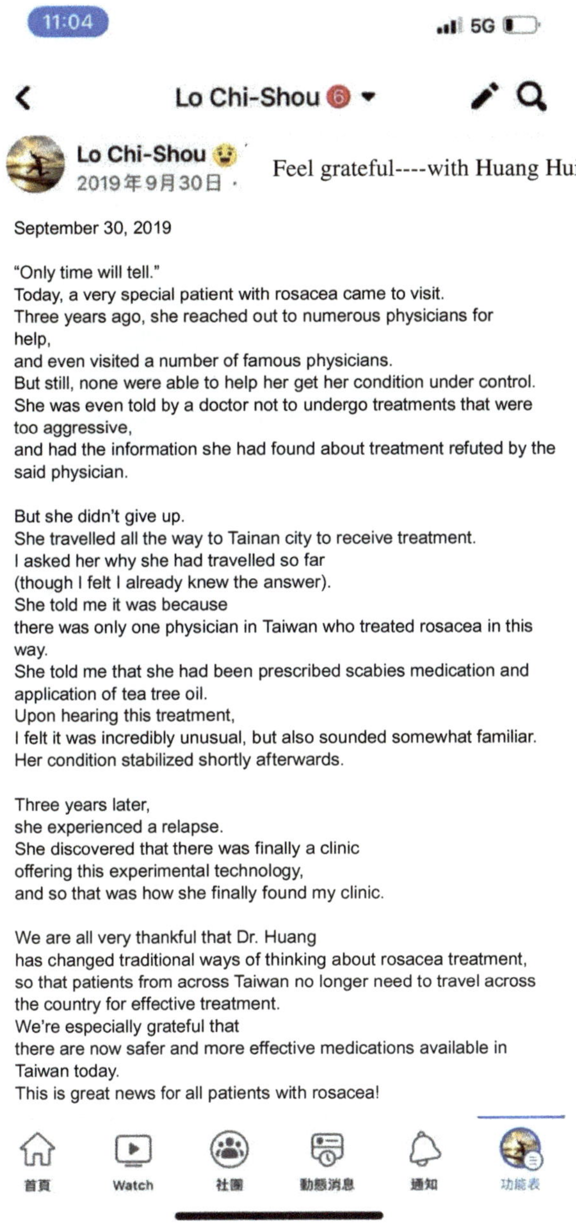

11:04 5G

Lo Chi-Shou 6

Lo Chi-Shou
2019年9月30日 ·

Feel grateful----with Huang Hui-Peng

September 30, 2019

"Only time will tell."
Today, a very special patient with rosacea came to visit.
Three years ago, she reached out to numerous physicians for help,
and even visited a number of famous physicians.
But still, none were able to help her get her condition under control.
She was even told by a doctor not to undergo treatments that were too aggressive,
and had the information she had found about treatment refuted by the said physician.

But she didn't give up.
She travelled all the way to Tainan city to receive treatment.
I asked her why she had travelled so far
(though I felt I already knew the answer).
She told me it was because
there was only one physician in Taiwan who treated rosacea in this way.
She told me that she had been prescribed scabies medication and application of tea tree oil.
Upon hearing this treatment,
I felt it was incredibly unusual, but also sounded somewhat familiar.
Her condition stabilized shortly afterwards.

Three years later,
she experienced a relapse.
She discovered that there was finally a clinic
offering this experimental technology,
and so that was how she finally found my clinic.

We are all very thankful that Dr. Huang
has changed traditional ways of thinking about rosacea treatment,
so that patients from across Taiwan no longer need to travel across the country for effective treatment.
We're especially grateful that
there are now safer and more effective medications available in Taiwan today.
This is great news for all patients with rosacea!

首頁 Watch 社團 動態消息 通知 功能表

**Figure 31.** Dr. Lo Chi-Shou provided a Facebook screenshot proving that, at that time, Dr. Huang was the only doctor in Taiwan who treated rosacea with antiparasitic drugs (2012–2017).

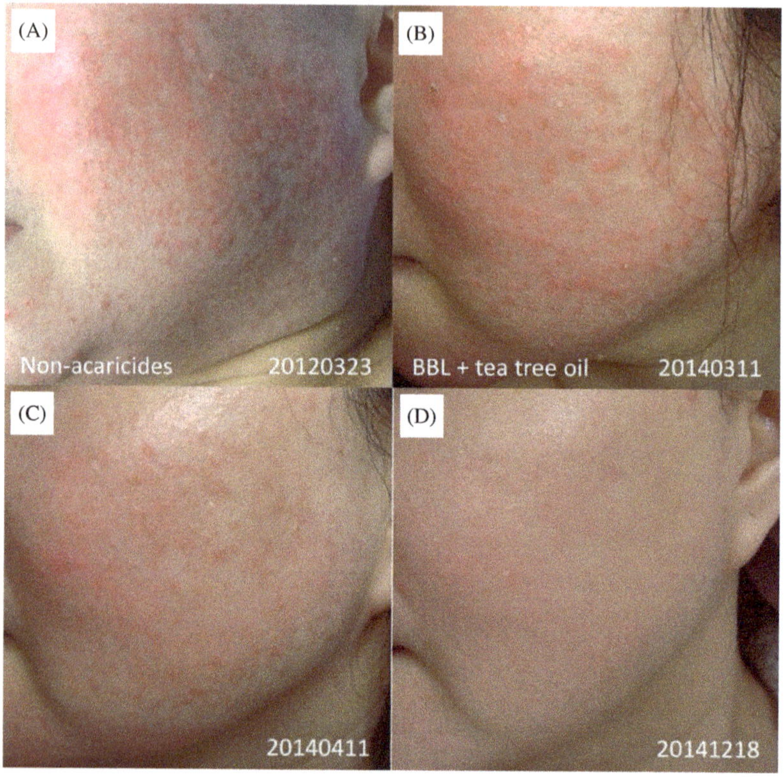


**Figure 32.** Sequential clinical photographs of a patient with papulopustular rosacea. The patient received conventional treatments for two years without improvement and experienced progressive worsening. After initiation of antiparasitic therapy (BBL combined with tea tree oil), the skin gradually improved and became clear of papulopustules.

on the skin is normal flora," "why antiparasitic drugs are required for rosacea," "nonsense and misleading," or "frightening words to scare people." A polite doctor will answer the patient noncommittally with a smile.

In the ROSCO conference by the Taiwanese Dermatology Association in 2015, I was nominated as one of the consensus members. During the conference, I mentioned some of my clinical observations on *Demodex* and rosacea. Unfortunately, most consensus members at that time agreed that *Demodex* played a role in rosacea, but they did not agree with the use of antiparasitic drugs to treat rosacea. In 2022, a patient relayed a conversation with a physician discussing a dermatologist's comment on

*Demodex* as "a hoax." At the time, I already had given dozens of speeches and workshops. We have consistently adhered to a path that is beneficial to patients, and we hope to see more friends, including doctors and patients with rosacea, will join to witness this path.

In 2013, our clinic began to examine every patient with rosacea for *Demodex* mites using a SSSB proposed by Forton.

In addition, we also developed the superficial needle-scraping for pustules and the TSM. In 2017, during the annual meeting organized by the Taiwanese Dermatological Association, we presented our practices in examination and treatment for rosacea and *Demodex* for the first time. As of 2022, we have made oral presentations and published papers on the efficacy of antiparasitic drugs and nonparasitic treatments for erythematous rosacea, flushing, PPR, and special types of rosacea.

These include studies on antiparasitic drugs in different dosages, exacerbation reactions, and its prevention methods. In my lecture in 2017, I anticipated that within 10 years, the treatment of *Demodex* in rosacea would become a fundamental skill for every dermatologist. Now, the achievement rate of this goal should be over 50%, and the widespread adoption is likely due to the fact that every dermatologist can replicate good treatment outcomes as long as they have the correct diagnosis and understand the key aspects of the treatment methods.

## 2.4 Methods of examining *Demodex*

### 2.4.1 *Superficial needle-scraping method*

We developed a new method to examine *Demodex* and named it the superficial needle-scraping for pustules. Prof. Lee Yu-Yun, Prof. Hsu Chao-Kai, and I published the study in the Journal of Cosmetic Dermatology, entitled "A new superficial needle-scraping method for assessing *Demodex* density in papulopustular rosacea."[1] In this study, we enrolled 40 patients with PPR and 35 patients with acne vulgaris, as a control group. These 35 patients with acne had no erythema, telangiectases, flushing, itching, or other symptoms of rosacea on their faces. The examination method was to use the outer convex end of an 18-gauge needle to scrape the contents of the pustule in a nearly horizontal manner. During the extraction process, the assisting hand must gently pinch the skin around the pustule, allowing the pustule to bulge slightly. After the contents of the pustule are extracted, the sample is placed on a glass slide and the procedure is repeated five times. Next, a drop of saline or tap water is added and the glass slide is covered with a coverslip, and *Demodex* mites are observed under a microscope for counting (Figure 33).

We used receiver operating characteristic (ROC) curve analysis, where the maximum value of the Youden index was used as the diagnostic criteria for the diagnostic standard. Simultaneously, we applied the SSSB on the 40 patients with PPR to compare the results of the two methods. The results showed no statistical differences in age and sex between the rosacea and acne groups; 33 out of 40 patients with PPR were found with *Demodex*, accounting for 83%.

In the acne group, only 5 out of 35 cases were found with *Demodex* (14%). The area under the ROC curve for this statistical analysis was 0.89, indicating that it is a highly effective method for distinguishing between high and low levels of *Demodex*. The DMD of the PPR group was 5.6 ± 4.2 mites/5 pustules, and the DMD of the acne group was 0.3 ± 1.0 mites/5 pustules ($p < 0.001$) (Figure 34).

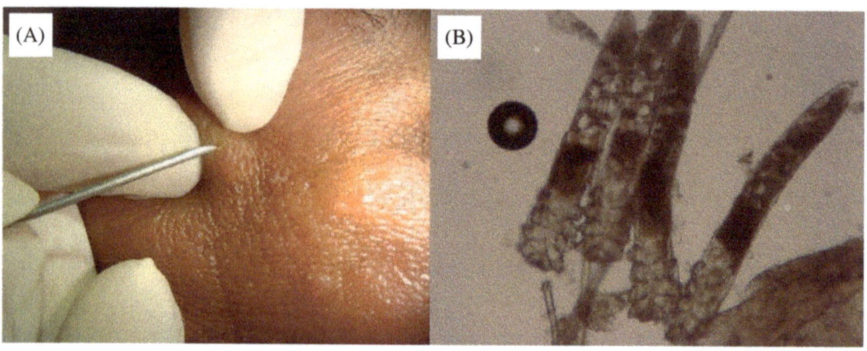


**Figure 33.** The superficial needle-scraping method was used to examine *Demodex*. (A) The contents of pustules were extracted with the bevel of an 18-gauge needle. *Demodex* mites were found under the microscope (B). Reference: Huang HP, Hsu CK, Lee JY. A new superficial needle-scraping method for assessing *Demodex* density in papulopustular rosacea. *J Cosmet Dermatol*. 2020;19(4):896–900.

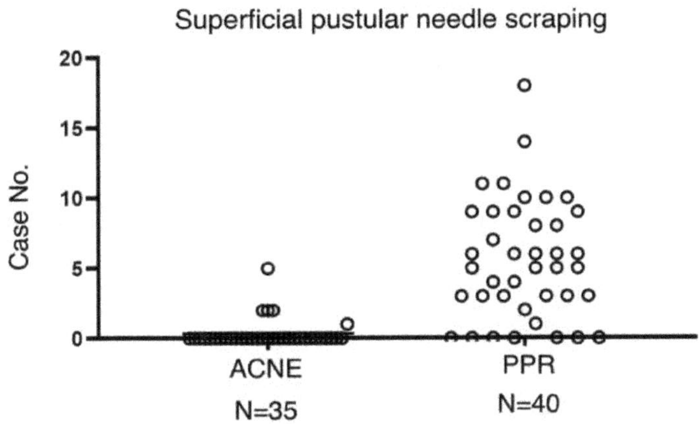


**Figure 34.** The superficial needle-scraping method was used to examine *Demodex*. The *Demodex* density of the papulopustular rosacea (PPR) group was 5.6 ± 4.2/5 pustules, and that of the acne group was 0.3 ± 1.0/5 pustules ($p < 0.001$).

We set the *Demodex* density of 3 mites/5 pustules as the diagnostic criteria to distinguish excessive from normal *Demodex* numbers. This method has a sensitivity of 0.78 and a specificity of 0.97 (Figure 35). Increasing the criteria to 6 mites/5 pustules increases the specificity to 100%. Regarding the SSSB on the 40 patients with PPR, the results showed that the DMD was 0–102/cm$^2$, with an average value of 8.4/cm$^2$. With a density over 6 mites/cm$^2$ as the diagnostic criteria, only 15 cases were positive, showing a sensitivity of 0.38.

The reasons for taking samples from five pustules in this study are (1) to save the examination time and (2) some patients have a limited number of pustules. When ten pustules are sampled, the diagnostic criteria should be ≥6 mites/10 pustules in proportion to the sampling size. Another advantage of the superficial needle-scraping method is that it can more directly disclose the association between pustules and mites. This examination method is suitable for patients with a high density of pustules on their faces (Figure 36). A limitation of the superficial needle-scraping method is that when the pustules disappear after treatment, we can no longer track DMD using this method.

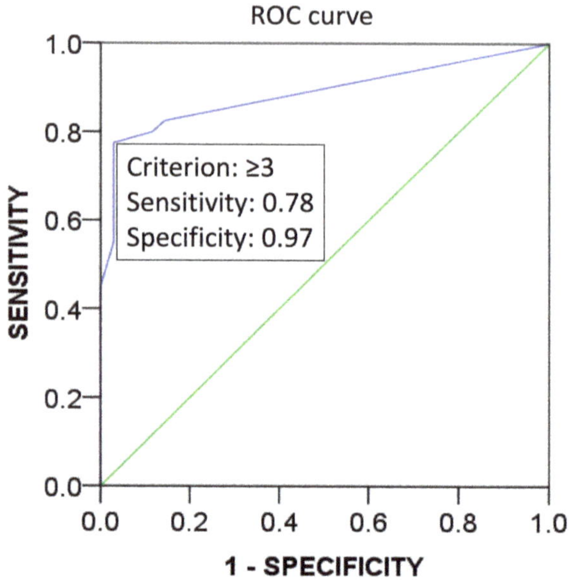


**Figure 35.** Receiver operating characteristic (ROC) curve of the groups receiving the superficial needle-scraping method. When the criterion was set at ≥3 mites/5 pustules, the sensitivity was 0.78, and the specificity was 0.97. Reference: Huang HP, Hsu CK, Lee JY. A new superficial needle-scraping method for assessing *Demodex* density in papulopustular rosacea. *J Cosmet Dermatol.* 2020;19(4):896–900.

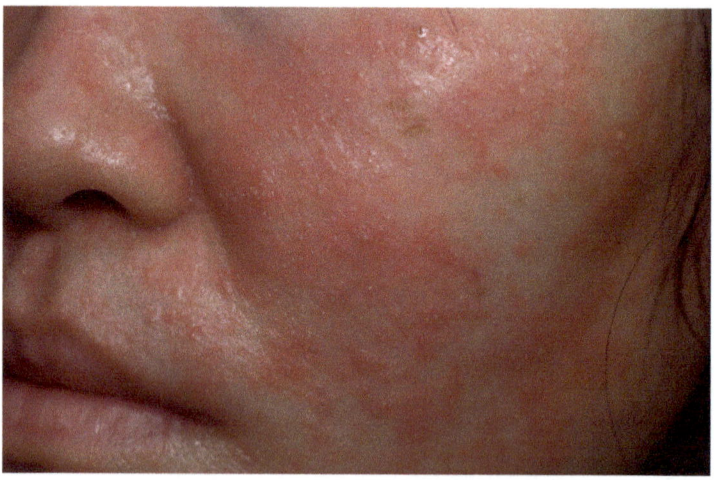

**Figure 36.** Demodex examination using the superficial needle-scraping method revealed 25 *Demodex* mites from five pustules.

### 2.4.2 *Thumbnail-squeezing method*

Because the superficial needle-scraping method to examine *Demodex* was only suitable for patients who were still in the pustule stage, we used the SSSB (Figure 37) for fairly a year to further diagnose and follow-up on those patients' treatment outcomes. However, the sensitivity of SSSB is too low, where very few *Demodex* mites are detected. Besides, there is a waiting time for the glue to dry, and during microscopy, many attempts involving different focal lengths on one hair may be required when a high level of *Demodex* mites is detected, making the SSSB method time-consuming.

Subsequently, we proposed an innovative method to examine *Demodex*, namely, the thumbnail-squeezing method (TSM).[2] The theoretical basis of this examination method is that *D. folliculorum* infests the superficial layer of hair follicles, namely the infundibulum in the follicular histology. *Demodex* mites infest hair follicles in an upside-down manner, with their tails at the orifice of the hair follicles. The body length of mites is 0.3 mm for adults and 0.4 mm for nymphs; therefore, as long as the squeezing depth is 0.5 mm, it is deep enough to collect mites for observation (Figure 38). We recruited 49 patients with ETR, 53 patients with PPR, and 49 healthy cases for the control group. The diagnostic criteria for rosacea are based on the ROSCO consensus. Patients had persistent centrofacial erythema and facial flushing caused by contributing factors. None of the patients had used antiparasitic drugs within 6 months. We marked a 1-$cm^2$ square on the face, mainly on the cheeks or other places where

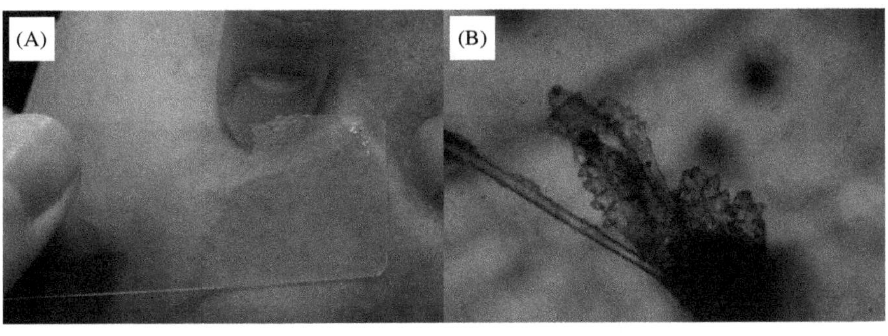


**Figure 37.** Standardized skin surface biopsy features application of quick-drying glue to stick the skin surface tissue (A). *Demodex* mites and hairs under the microscope (B).

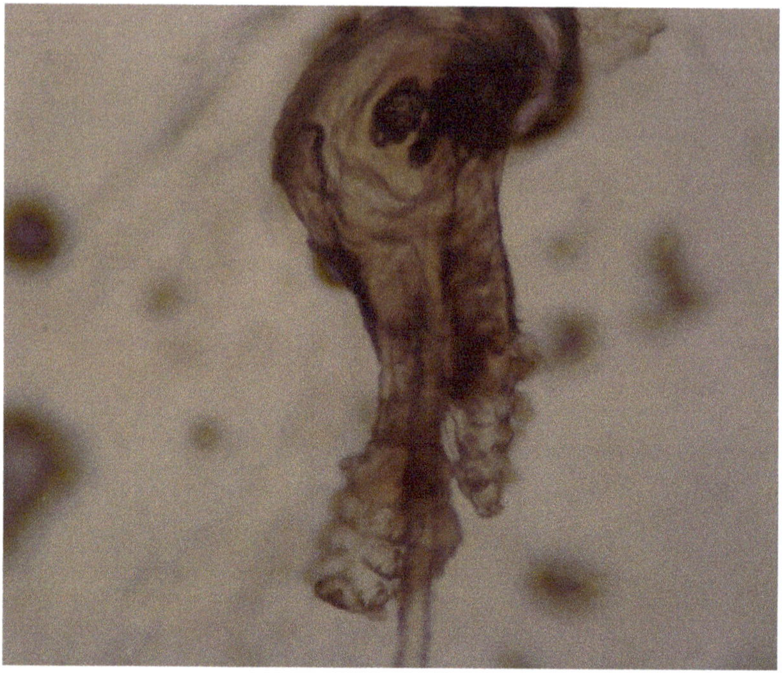

**Figure 38.** Standardized skin surface biopsy shows that *D. folliculorum* infest hair follicles in an upside-down manner, with their tails at the orifice of the hair follicles. The body length of mites is 0.3–0.4 mm; therefore, as long as the squeezing depth is 0.5 mm, it is deep enough to collect mites for observation.

mites are abundant, such as the glabella, chin, and nose. We also tried to avoid areas with dense pustules or skin swelling. The person who took samples wore gloves that fit the hands and could hold them tightly. Some mineral oil could be applied to the sampling site to lubricate and soften the contents of the hair follicles.

The assisting hand of the sampler was used to stretch, pinch, or hold the skin of the sampling site, where the distal free end of the thumbnail that is used to squeeze needs to be 1–2 mm long to squeeze the skin to a depth of 0.5 mm. The thumb repeatedly squeezed and released the skin and advanced within this 1-cm$^2$ area, advancing 1–2 mm each time. The contents squeezed out from hair follicles would automatically stick to the tightly held gloves, and we transferred the contents obtained from this 1 cm$^2$ of skin to a glass slide. Because the tissue sticks to the glove on convex curved surface of the thumb, the squeezed-out contents can be transferred entirely to the glass slide without a loss. Finally, we added a drop of mineral oil to the sample and observed the glass slide under a microscope to count the number of mites (https://youtu.be/a9S6cvfHX78?si=k-YRjMRXNJ7KeOBf).

Under a microscope, we spread out the specimen and were able to clearly observe *Demodex* mites at different stages: eggs, larvae, protonymphs, nymphs, and adults, as well as count the number of *Demodex* mites of each stage. The mite densities of patients with ETR and PPR were higher than those in the control group.

The mean ± standard error of the three groups was 105 ± 16.9/cm$^2$, 106 ± 14.6/cm$^2$, and 7.8 ± 2.8/cm$^2$, respectively. The areas under ROC curves of the ETR group and the PPR group were both 0.95. With a density >11 mites/cm$^2$ as the diagnostic criteria, the sensitivity of both ETR and PPR is 92%, and the specificity is 90% (Figure 39). This study was jointly published by Prof. Lee Yu-Yun, Prof. Hsu Chao-Kai, and I in Journal of the European Academy of Dermatology and Venereology.[2]

Junior practitioners may make mistakes in some aspects such as (1) not having nails long enough to apply adequate deep pressure, (2) gloves not fit enough to squeeze and collect samples, and (3) thumbs not forceful

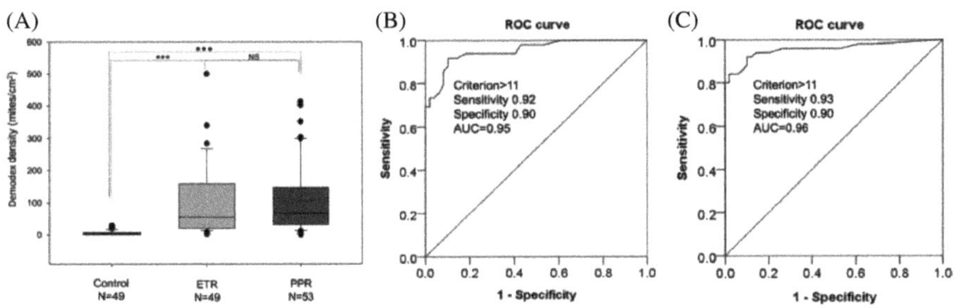


**Figure 39.** Thumbnail-squeezing method. (A) The ETR and PPR patient groups have higher *Demodex* density than the control group, with the values of 105 ± 16.9/cm$^2$ (mean ± standard error), 106 ± 14.6/cm$^2$, and 7.8 ± 2.8/cm$^2$, respectively. (B, C) The areas under the ROC curves of the ETR group and the PPR group were both 0.95. With a density >11 mites/cm$^2$ as the cut-off value, the sensitivity of both ETR and PPR is 92%, and the specificity is 90%. Reference: Huang HP, Hsu CK, Lee JY. Thumbnail-squeezing method: an effective method for assessing *Demodex* density in rosacea. *J Eur Acad Dermatol Venereol.* 2020;34(7):e343-e345.

enough where the application of hands and finger muscles requires learning and accommodation. Generally, the first attempt is to learn the maneuver, the practice on the second day is to review and learn the coordination of hand muscles, and the practice on the third day and onward is to strengthen hand muscles. After 2 weeks of practice, all practitioners should be able to excel in this method. The recommended location for sampling is the skin manifestations shown in Figures 11 and 12 of the demodicosis spectrum, where areas of intensely inflamed skin should be avoided. The assisting hand should be best utilized to hold the skin for sampling. The squeezing pressure should be even and gentle. Moreover, attention should be paid to the fragile skin of patients who have been applying steroids and taking retinoic acid for a long time and are prone to skin tears and bruises.

The TSM is a very effective method for determining DMD and observing mite forms. We have the microphotographs of *D. folliculorum* arranged as per their lifecycle from the eggs, larvae, protonymphs, and nymphs to adults, which is rare and valuable (Figure 40). *Demodex* brevis is also easy to sample (Figure 41).

Because *D. brevis* mainly lives in sebaceous glands, particularly near the sebaceous ducts, the squeezing depth of 0.5 mm exceeds the depth of the sebaceous ducts. This examination can be performed on any part of the face, whether a convex or concave surface. As long as the skin can be held tightly and squeezed, the skin other than the face, such as the neck, chest, and scalp, can also be sampled for examination. Diagnostic criteria should be slightly lowered on samples collected from parts other than the face. There are a lot of hairs on the scalp. It should be moisturized with mineral oil before the examination. The technique is shown in Figures 42 and 43.

### 2.4.3 *How to select a suitable examination method?*

We believe that each method for sampling *Demodex* has its own advantages (Table 4), and it is recommended to choose the appropriate method according to the condition.

I. Thumbnail-squeezing method (TSM)[2] (modified thumb squeezing method): It features the use of a marking pen to draw a 1-$cm^2$ square on the face (Figure 44) and is suitable for any lesion or sampling site. Its

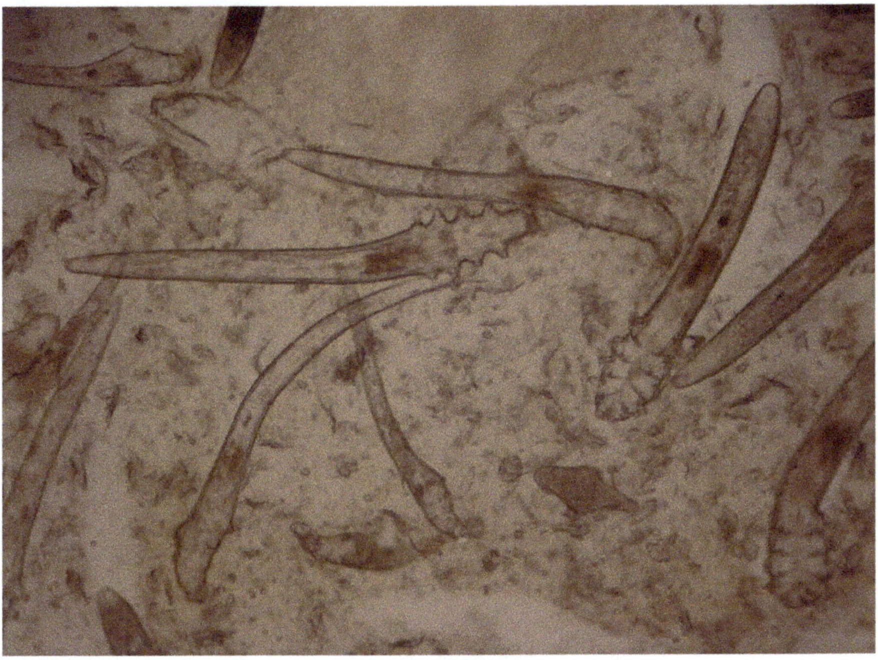

**Figure 40.** Lifecycle of *D. folliculorum* from the eggs, larvae, protonymphs, and nymphs to adults. Reference: Huang HP, Hsu CK, Lee JY. Thumbnail-squeezing method: an effective method for assessing *Demodex* density in rosacea. *J Eur Acad Dermatol Venereol.* 2020;34(7):e343-e345.

advantages include convenience in counting the number of mites; intact mites collected; high detection rate of *Demodex*, including *Demodex brevis*; and time-saving. Practitioners need to practice the technique, excel in the force, and be careful to avoid injuring the skin. The diagnostic criteria is >11 mites/cm$^2$. The sensitivity of this method to ETR and PPR is 0.92, and the specificity is 0.9. This is the most frequently used method in our clinic. It is quick, accurate, convenient, and without pungent smell from the quick-drying glue. Squeezing can also be done in a gentle way, and the process from collecting to counting the number of mites only takes 1–2 minutes.

II. Superficial needle-scraping for pustules (SNS)[1] is suitable for cases with pustules and severe inflammation and provides more straightforward evidence of *Demodex* mites and pustules, with a sensitivity of

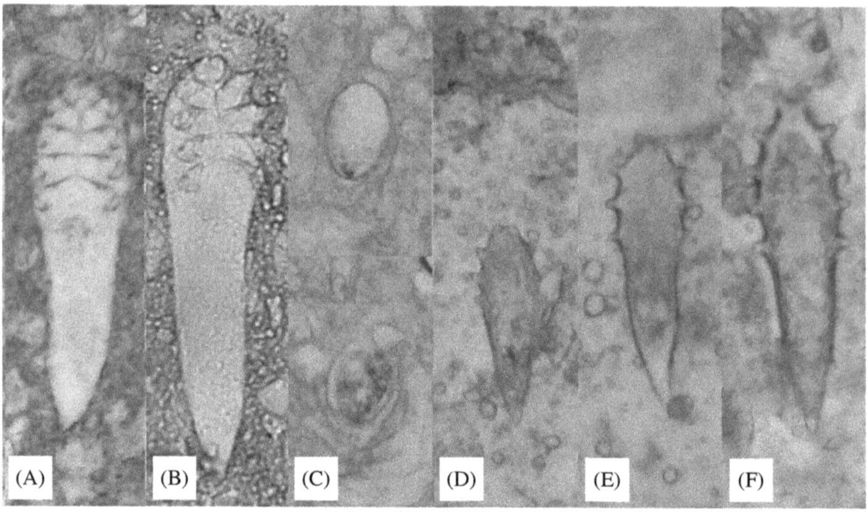


**Figure 41.** Morphology of *D. brevis* from left to right: adult (A,B), egg (C), larvae (D), protonymph (E), and nymph (F).

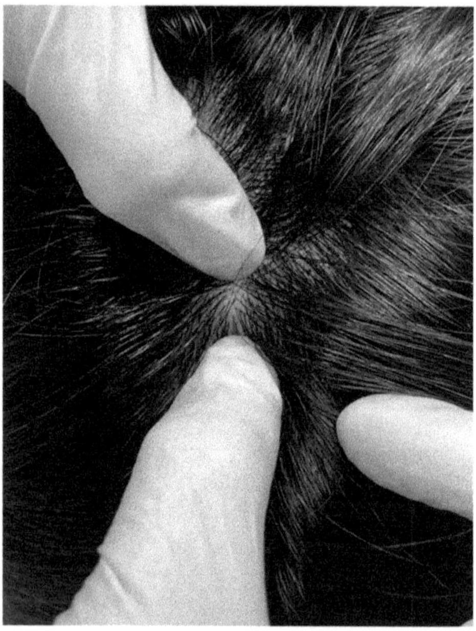

**Figure 42.** When the thumbnail-squeezing method is used on the scalp, two thumbs face each other, where one thumb is fixed and the other squeezes.

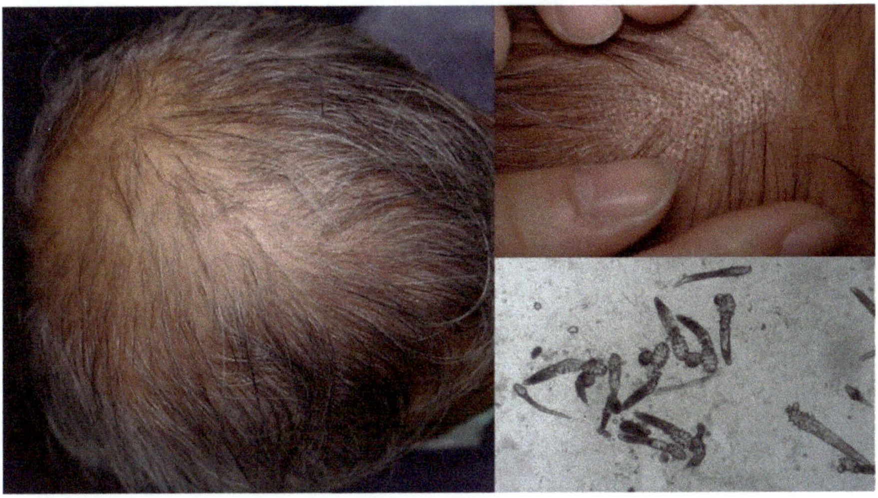

**Figure 43.** The male patient complained of scalp itching and had enlarged pores. The result of the TSM showed excessive *Demodex* density.

0.78 and a specificity of 0.97. One disadvantage of SNS is that follow-up on mites will become challenging once the pustules clear up. For patients with dense pustules, such as the one in Figure 37, the SNS method is the best option.

III. Two consecutive SSSB (1 + 2)[3]: Prof. Forton has proposed a new version of this technique of conducting SSSB twice consecutively. Before sampling, the skin and glass slides are cleaned with ether. The diagnostic criteria are as follows: the first sample is >5 mites/cm$^2$, the second sample >10 mites/cm$^2$, and the total >15 mites/cm$^2$. For PPR, the sensitivity of this method is 0.985, and the specificity is 0.97. The SSSB 1 + 2 method is good and suitable for all patients. In my view, the disadvantages of this method are as follows: the sampling site is limited by the slide shape, as some parts are not easy for sampling. Additionally, in cases with a large number of *Demodex* mites, counting can be time-consuming.

IV. Reflectance confocal microscopy (RCM)[4]: The sensitivity of this method for ETR and PPR is 0.82, and the specificity is 0.8. This method requires an advanced instrument, which is expensive, making it hard to be widely applied.

**Table 4.** Summary of Methods to Examine Demodex

| Method | Thumbnail-squeezing method | Two consecutive standardized skin surface biopsies | Reflectance confocal microscopy | Superficial needle-scraping method |
|---|---|---|---|---|
| Rosacea subtypes | ETR, PPR | PPR | ETR, PPR | PPR |
| Diagnostic criteria | > 11 mites/cm$^2$ | (1) > 5, (2) > 10, and (1+2) > 15 mites/cm$^2$ | > 0.17 mites/follicle | > 2 mites/5 pustules |
| Sensitivity | 0.92 | 0.985 | 0.82 | 0.78 |
| Specificity | 0.90 | 0.97 | 0.8 | 0.97 |
| Note | Squeezing depth 0.5 mm | Cleanse skin with ether | Assessment area 10 mm$^2$ | Sample 5 pustules |
| Advantages | Suitable for all cases and sampling sites; noninvasive; time-saving; easy to observe because of the spreading out of mites; applicable to both kinds of *Demodex* mites in the five stages of the lifecycle for morphology, different forms, activity, and enumeration of mites. | Noninvasive | Noninvasive | Directly reveal the association between pustules and *Demodex* |

(*Continued*)

**Table 4.** (*Continued*)

| Method | Thumbnail-squeezing method | Two consecutive standardized skin surface biopsies | Reflectance confocal microscopy | Superficial needle-scraping method |
|---|---|---|---|---|
| Disadvantages | Painful, red marks over squeezing sites | The sampling site may be limited by the slide shape as some parts are not easy to apply; it may be relatively more time-consuming to sample and count when the number of *Demodex* mites is large. Pungent smells from the glue. | Expensive, making it hard to be widely applied. | Invasive, only applicable for pustules. |
| Author | Huang Hui-Peng, Hsu Chao-Kai, and Lee Yu-Yun | Forton FM, De Maertelaer V | Turgut EA et al | Huang Hui-Peng, Hsu Chao-Kai, and Lee Yu-Yun |

Note: ETR: erythematotelangiectatic rosacea; PPR: papulopustular rosacea.

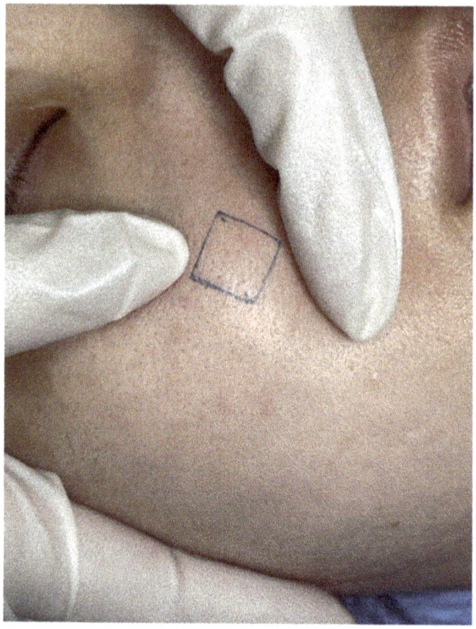

**Figure 44.** The thumbnail-squeezing method for sampling the skin at the size of 1 $cm^2$.

## 2.5 Classification of demodicosis

According to the original classification by Ayres, demodicosis is classified into pityriasis folliculorum (1930) and rosacea-like demodicosis (1963). Later, variations such as abscess and perioral dermatitis were published.

In 2014, a new classification system was proposed by Prof. Chen Wen-Jie and Prof. Plewig, where demodicosis was classified into two forms, with variations including spinulate demodicosis, papulopustular demodicosis, perioral demodicosis, periorbital demodicosis, periauricular demodicosis, and nodulocystic/conglobate demodicosis (Table 5).[5]

Dr. Huang Hui-Peng propose that the clinical manifestations of demodicosis of the skin can be classified into papulopustular demodicosis and nonpapulopustular demodicosis. The former can be papule only or papulopustules. Skin lesions of those with papules can be at a size as small as a pinpoint, pinhead, or plaques when multiple lesions are fused together. Those with papulopustules may have skin lesions as large as a pinpoint, pinhead, or nodule cyst (Figure 11). Skin lesions of nonpapulopustular demodicosis may develop large pores and/or follicular plugs.

**Table 5.** Human demodicosis: proposed classification and nomenclature

| **Huang's classification** | **Huang's description** | **W. Chen and G. Plewig's nomenclature*** | **Ordinary terminology*** |
|---|---|---|---|
| Papulopustular demodicosis | 1. Papulopustules<br>2. Papules | 1. Papulopustular demodicosis, perioral, periorbital and periauricular demodicosis<br>2. Nodulocystic/ conglobate demodicosis | 1. Rosacea-like demodicosis,<br>2. Perioral (periorificial) demodicosis<br>3. *Demodex* abscess |
| Non-papulopustular demodicosis | 1. Large pores (orange skin-like appearance, large tan-colored pores)<br>2. Follicular scale (Frosted appearance, sandpaper-like appearance)<br>3. Large pores + follicular plugs (Nutmeg grater appearance) | Spinulate demodicosis | Pityriasis folliculorum<br>1. Frosted appearance<br>2. Sandpaper-like appearance<br>3. Nutmeg grater appearance |

*, Reference 5.

They can also develop large tan-colored pores formed by enlarged pores, orange skin-like appearance, protruding white spicule-like follicular scales with frosted or sandpaper-like appearance defined by granularity, and the coexistence of enlarged pores and white follicular plugs with nutmeg grater appearance (Figure 12). Among them, the signs of large tan-colored pores formed by enlarged pores and orange skin-like appearance were not reported in previous studies. The reason for classifying papulopustular demodicosis into papulopustular and papular is that the treatment of the latter is more difficult, which will be discussed in detail later in Section 3.3.8.2.

## 2.6 Eyelids could be a hotspot for *Demodex* in infants and children

Where does *Demodex* in infants and young children come from? What are the symptoms of demodicosis in children? We had a 21-month-old patient who had a recurring sty. From one eyelash sample, we spotted three *D. folliculorum*, and they were very well developed. However, the mites we collected from the child's nose did not develop very well. Compared with those from the eyes, the mites from the nose were smaller in length and width, and their body size was almost only a fourth of that of the mites at the eyes (Figure 45).

Another patient, who was 5 years and 9 months old, had a recurring sty during her ages of 4 and 5 years. Later, her sty disappeared, and small pustules began to appear on her nose, which lasted for a year. After another year, the child had obvious persistent erythema on her face (Figure 46). *Demodex* mites require sebum or meibum to survive; however, they also feed on epidermal cells of follicles. Newborns should be free from *Demodex* at the time of birth. Through close contact with the faces of adults, particularly mothers, *Demodex* mites may crawl onto their faces. At this time, androgen level is low, and the development of the sebaceous glands is not complete. It should not be easy for mites to obtain

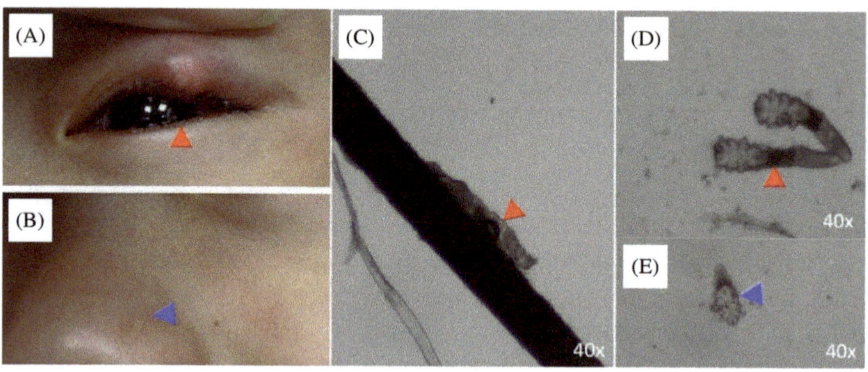


**Figure 45.** Demodicosis in children manifested by a recurring hordeolum in a 21-month-old child (A), with healthy skin on the face (B), where three mites were found on one eyelash sample and were well developed (C, D), whereas mites collected at the nose were poorly developed (E). Compared with the mites from the eyes, the mites from the nose were smaller in length and width, and their body size was almost only a fourth of that of the mites at the eyes (E). Arrows indicate the sampling sites and *Demodex* mites, respectively.

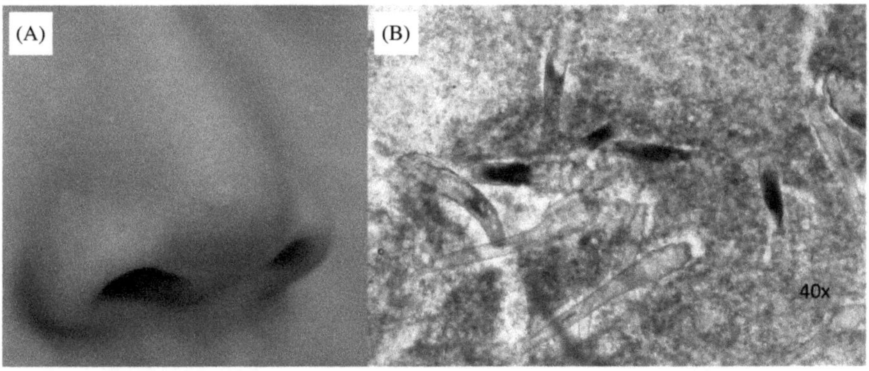


**Figure 46.** A girl patient, who was 5 years and 9 months old, had a recurring sty during her age 4–5 year. Later, her sty disappeared, and small pustules (A) began to appear on her nose, which lasted for a year, with the mite density on her nose being 50 mites/cm$^2$ (B). After another year, the child had obvious persistent erythema on her face.

sufficient sebum on their face. However, the meibomian glands of children's eyelids are already very fully developed, and the meibomian glands are almost at their best function when they are born. Therefore, the *Demodex* mites that infest the eyelids in early childhood develop better and are larger than the mites that infest the face (Figure 47). After puberty, androgen begins to be produced, stimulating the development of sebaceous glands. At this time, the face provides enough nutrients for *Demodex* to develop well. Clinically, demodicosis on the eye lashes and face can occur simultaneously or separately. The youngest patients with demodicosis in our clinic were 3 years and 1 month old on the face and 1 year and 9 months old on the eyelashes, respectively. The examination method in children for *Demodex* mites is to gently pick the affected skin with the index finger nail to take a sample while wearing a glove.

## 2.7 Experiences of using ivermectin cream that has antiparasitic and anti-inflammatory effects in Taiwan

In 2015, Taieb et al. reported that topical ivermectin cream 1% is more effective than metronidazole cream 0.75% in treating inflammatory lesions of rosacea.[6] After reading this article, I repeatedly suggested that pharmaceutical suppliers introduced this drug to Taiwan as soon as possible

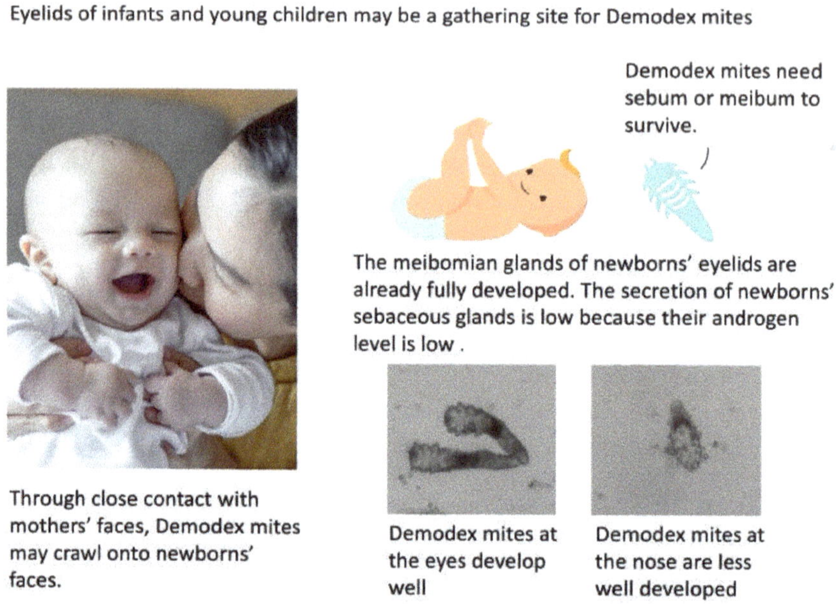


**Figure 47.** Through close contact with mothers' faces, *Demodex* mites may crawl onto newborns' faces. Infants' androgen levels are low, and the development of the sebaceous glands is incomplete. However, the meibomian glands of newborns' eyelids are already fully developed. Therefore, the *Demodex* mites that infest the eyelids in early childhood develop better and are larger than those that infest the face.

to benefit patients with rosacea. In 2017, after the pharmaceutical supplier informed me that they had submitted the drug for approval to the FDA, I immediately suggested that the Department of Dermatology of the National Cheng Kung University Hospital introduced this drug on a special project. Once the drug was available, I immediately referred 30 patients to the National Cheng Kung University Hospital in a month to get ivermectin cream 1% treatment and followed up on their conditions and treatment outcomes. With preliminary experience and clinical data, I presented first-hand information on the use of ivermectin cream 1% in Taiwan at a dinner hosted by the supplier at the annual Meeting of the Taiwanese Dermatological Association (Figure 48).

From April to September 2017, 33 patients were recruited. Excluding 10 cases with whom we lost contact during their follow-up and dropped

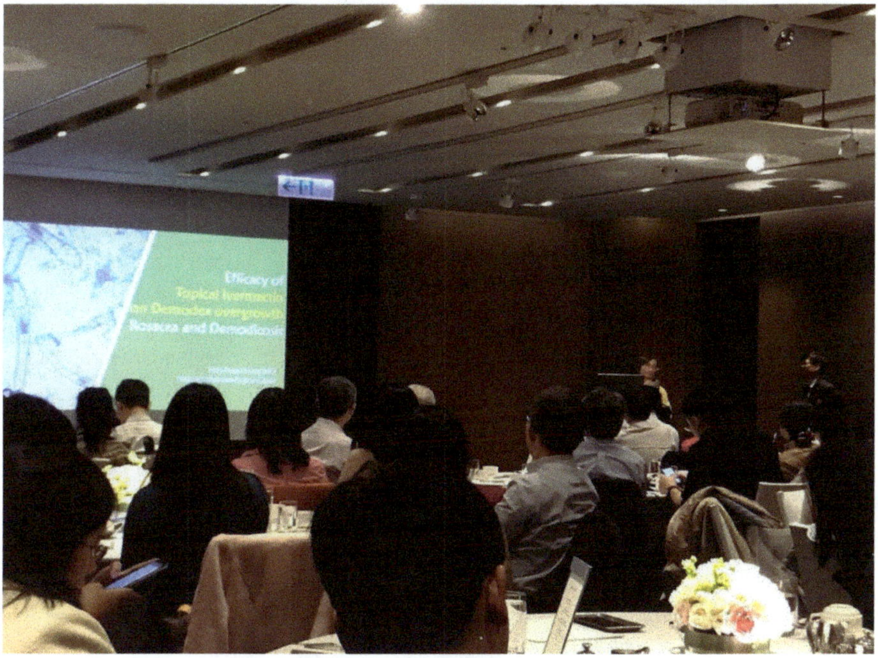

**Figure 48.** During the 2017 Annual Meeting of the Taiwanese Dermatological Association, Dr. Hui-Peng Huang reported using antiparasitic therapy to treat patients with rosacea and excessive *Demodex* mites. This was first-hand information on the use of ivermectin cream 1% in Taiwan. At that time, the chairperson of the dinner was Prof. Lee Yu-Yun from the Department of Dermatology of the National Cheng Kung University Hospital.

out midway, the 23 cases included 17 patients with ETR and 6 patients with primary demodicosis. The patients with ETR were classified into 5 grades, 0 to 4, according to the CEA, where 12 of the 17 patients (71%) experienced 1–2 CEA grades of improvement in their erythema on the face (Figures 49 and 50). I remember that the doctors attending the dinner were very enthusiastic. There were >90 attendees in total. The response and discussion were also very lively. This was the beginning of Taiwan's dermatology community re-examining the relationship between *Demodex* and rosacea and using antiparasitic therapy to treat patients with rosacea and excessive *Demodex* mites, which is an important milestone.

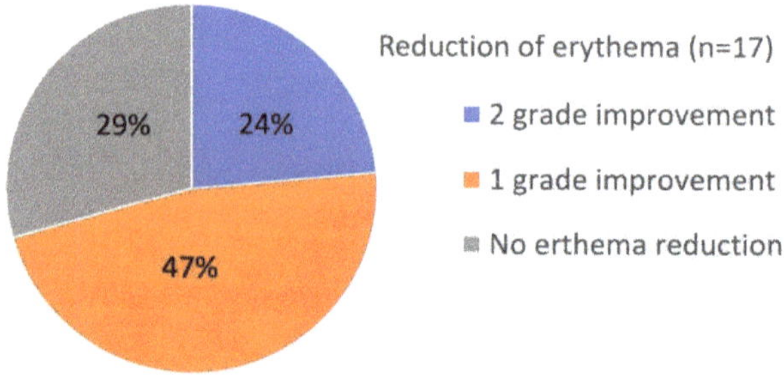


**Figure 49.** For those who were treated with ivermectin cream 1%, 12 of the 17 patients (71%) were found with 1 to 2 CEA grades of improvement in their erythema on the face.

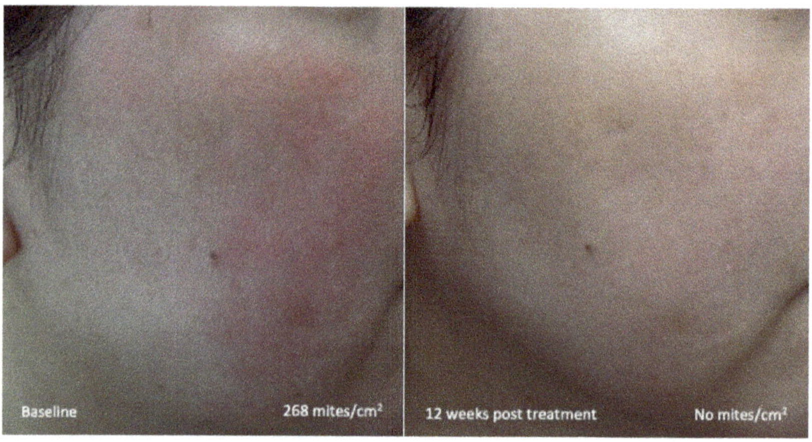


**Figure 50.** Patients with rosacea who were treated with ivermectin cream 1% and oral carvedilol for 12 weeks showed that their CEA grade remained at 1 and *Demodex* mites were undetectable.

## 2.8 Analysis of 80 rosacea cases

Subsequently, we treated more patients. We statistically analyzed the clinical results of a total of 80 patients with ETR and PPR combined with excessive *Demodex* mites from April 2017 to December 2018, who were treated with ivermectin 1% cream alone or in combination with other drugs. The patient numbers and the drug combinations are as follows: 47 cases of carvedilol 6.25 mg two to three times a day, 42 cases of levocetirizine 6 mg daily, 3 cases of tacrolimus 0.1% ointment twice a day,

14 cases of isotretinoin 10 mg to 20 mg daily, 7 cases of doxycycline 100 mg daily, 6 cases of minocycline 100 mg daily, 11 cases of metronidazole 0.75% gel twice a day, and 7 cases of tranexamic acid (50 mg/mL) applied on the face daily. Three of the 80 patients discontinued their treatment because of papulopustular exacerbation. After 2–16 weeks of treatment, 37 (88%) of the 42 patients with ETR with a CEA $\geq 2$ could achieve successful treatment; only 24 of the 35 patients with PPR could achieve successful treatment, and the other 11 patients only made clinical improvement. Successful treatment was defined as the final CEA $\leq 1$ in patients with ETR and the complete or almost complete clearance of papules and pustules in patients with PPR. Further analysis of the total dosage and treatment duration of ivermectin 1% cream used in these two groups of patients with PPR revealed no statistically significant difference in the total dose between the two groups. The treatment duration was $8.0 \pm 3.8$ weeks (4–16 weeks) in the group with successful treatment and was $4.8 \pm 1.9$ weeks (2–8 weeks) in the group with clinical improvement, which showed a significant difference ($p < 0.001$; Figure 51). The *Demodex* densities in these two groups were significantly different before and after each treatment, but there was no significant difference between each other before and after treatment. However, the final *Demodex* density of the group with successful treatment was $7.5 \pm 2.2/cm^2$, and that of the group with clinical improvement was $23.4 \pm 10.7/cm^2$ (Figure 52). The TSM was used in this study, and the diagnostic criteria was 11 mites/$cm^2$.

We conclude that the extension of the treatment duration of ivermectin 1% cream and the final *Demodex* density dropping to a normal value can improve the treatment outcome in patients with PPR.

We observed an interesting aspect. Among the 80 patients with rosacea, 4 cases had a decrease in *D. folliculorum* and an increase in *D. brevis*, but there was no sign of clinical deterioration. For example, case number 32 had PPR, and his density ratio of *D. folliculorum* to *D. brevis* changed from 52:44/$cm^2$ before treatment to 10:230/$cm^2$ after treatment. Subsequently, after 2 weeks of taking 10-mg isotretinoin per day, the total number of *Demodex* mites finally dropped to two *D. brevis* mites/$cm^2$. Thus, we speculate that *D. brevis* plays a much less important role in causing a clinical disease than *D. folliculorum*. In our nearly 10 years of clinical experience, we had seen only one case with small pustules on

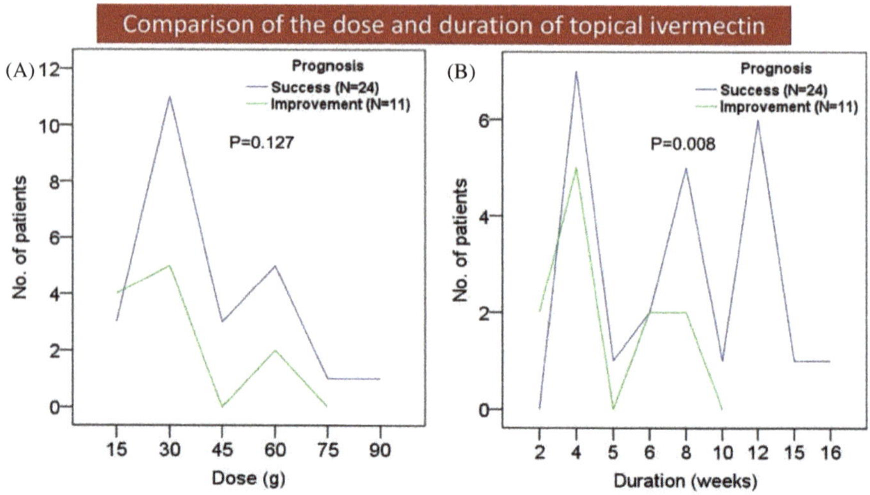


**Figure 51.** Patients with PPR were divided into two groups: the successful treatment group and the clinical improvement group. There was no statistically significant difference in the total dose of ivermectin 1% cream between the two groups. In terms of the treatment duration, it was 8.0 ± 3.8 weeks (4–16 weeks) in the successful treatment group and 4.8 ± 1.9 weeks (2–8 weeks) in the clinical improvement group, where a statistically significant difference was found ($p < 0.001$).

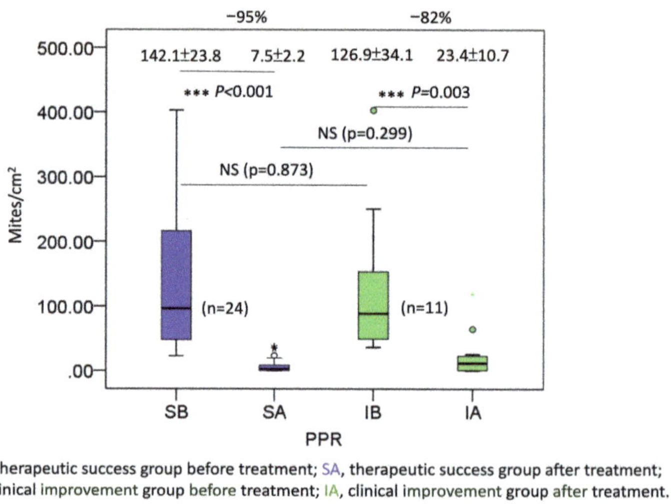


**Figure 52.** The final *Demodex* density in the successful treatment group of patients with PPR was 7.5 ± 2.2/cm$^2$, and that of the clinical improvement group was 23.4 ± 10.7/cm$^2$.

the face, who was found with only *D. brevis* via the superficial needle-scraping method and the TSM.

## 2.9 Report of a case–control study on treatments of ivermectin 1% cream and ivermectin 1% cream combined with oral carvedilol for rosacea erythema

This paper was authored by Huang Hui-Peng, Prof. Lee Yu-Yun, and Prof. Hsu Chao-Kai in Dermatologic Therapy (2021; 34: e14899).[7]

Some medical studies have confirmed that topical ivermectin 1% cream is effective in treating PPR,[6,8–10] but its effect on erythematous rosacea with high DMD has not been well documented. Thus, we retrospectively analyzed patients with erythematous rosacea and persistent centrofacial erythema who visited us from April 2017 to June 2018. We found that these patients also had excessive *Demodex* mites, which were assessed via the TSM, and the definition of excessive *Demodex* mites is a density >11 mites/cm$^2$. All patients showed CEA $\geq$ 2. The treatment received by the patients was ivermectin 1% cream at the amount equivalent to two knuckle lengths a day or oral carvedilol 6.25 mg twice a day. Some patients also took the oral antihistamine levocetirizine 5 mg to relieve itching. The CEA is divided into five grades from 0 to 4. The definition of erythema treatment response is: excellent, erythema is reduced by more than 1 CEA grade, and the final CEA = 1; good, the erythema is reduced by 1–2 CEA grades, and the final CEA is >1; fair, the scope of the erythema is reduced, but the CEA grade remains unchanged; and none, no improvement.

Our initial medical records were derived from the 80 patients with ETR and PPR combined with excessive *Demodex* mites described in the previous paragraph. Among them, 41 patients were excluded because of treatment with other drugs, including oral isotretinoin, antibiotic doxycycline, tacrolimus 0.1%, and metronidazole gel 0.75%.

Among the remaining 39 patients, 16 had PPR and 23 had ETR. Five patients had initial deterioration after treatment, because of which three of them stopped treatment. In four patients, the DMD increased after 1–4 weeks of treatment. Their CEA grades and DMD at the time when mite resistance was detected were also used for final analysis. In the end, there were 36 patients included, with their age- and sex-matched, where 14 of them received ivermectin 1% cream and the other 22 received ivermectin 1% cream and oral carvedilol (Table 6). The patients had a medical history of rosacea ranging from 1 month to 18 years, the treatment duration of ivermectin 1% cream was 1–12 weeks, and the total dose was 7–90 g. There were no significant differences in the treatment duration and total dose between the two groups.

Regarding treatment effects, overall, the two groups showed significant improvement in facial erythema (Figure 53), where 26 out of 36 cases (72%) achieved an excellent response, 2 cases had a good response, 4 cases had a fair response, and 4 cases had no improvement. The CEA grade of the ivermectin group was significantly reduced from 1.9 ± 0.7 to 1.1 ± 0.3 ($p < 0.01$), and that of the combined treatment group was significantly reduced from 2.2 ± 0.4 to 1.2 ± 0.4 ($p < 0.01$). The CEA grades before and after treatment and reductions in CEA grades showed no

**Table 6.** Clinical data of the 36 cases of rosacea (Source: *Dermatol Ther.* 2021; 34(2):e14899)

| | **IVM group** | **IVM-CAR group** |
|---|---|---|
| Case number | 14 (papulopustular 5) | 22 (papulopustular 8) |
| Age, years | 24–68 (42.3 ± 12.1)* | 22–61 ( 43.5 ± 11.3)* |
| Sex | 12 female, 2 male† | 21 female, 1 male† |
| Disease history | 1 month–10 years | 2 months to 18 years |
| CEA before and after treatment | 1.9 ± 0.67<br>1.1 ± 0.27 ($p < 0.01$) | 2.2 ± 0.39<br>1.2 ± 0.43 ($p < 0.01$) |
| IVM total dose | 7–90 g (27 ± 20)‡ | 15–60 g (37 ± 18)‡ |
| IVM treatment duration | 1–12 weeks§ | 3–10 weeks§ |
| Erythema response | Excellent 9 (64%) | Excellent 17 (77%) |
| *Demodex* density (mites/cm$^2$) | | |
| Before treatment | 120 ± 25.0 | 115 ± 23.0 |
| After treatment | 40.7 ± 15.2 ($p < 0.01$) | 28.0 ± 10.0 ($p < 0.01$) |

CEA, clinician's erythema assessment; IVM, ivermectin 1% cream; IVM-CAR, ivermectin 1% cream combined with oral carvedilol; excellent response, CEA reduction of at least 1 grade, and ultimately ≤1; *, $p = 0.707$; †, $p = 0.959$; ‡, $p = 0.951$; §, $p = 0.596$.

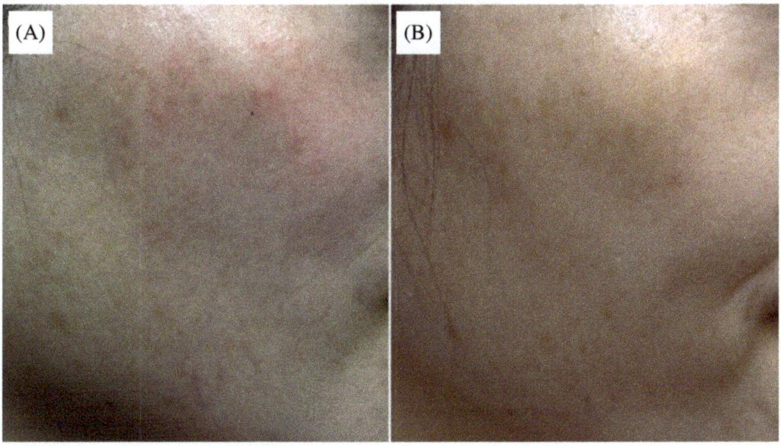


**Figure 53.** A female patient with rosacea (A) used 15 g of ivermectin cream alone for 4 weeks. After 6 months, the erythema on her face almost completely cleared up (B), and her *Demodex* density dropped from 31 mites/cm$^2$ to 10 mites/cm$^2$. Reference: *Dermatol Ther*. 2021; 34 (2): e14899.

significant difference between the two groups. Finally, 30 of 36 patients (83%) had CEA $\leq 1$, where 93% of the patients in the ivermectin group met this standard, and the percentage in the combined treatment group was 77%. Although there is no statistical correlation between CEA and DMD before treatment, there is a statistical correlation between their reductions after treatment (Spearman's rho = 0.50, $p = 0.002$) (Figure 54). The average DMD significantly decreased after treatment, and the values of the mean ± standard error of the two groups also significantly decreased from 120 ± 25.0 mites/cm$^2$ to 40.7 ± 15.2 mites/cm$^2$ and from 115 ± 23.0 mites/cm$^2$ to 28.0 ± 10.0 mites/cm$^2$, respectively. There was no significant difference between the two groups in DMDs before and after treatment.

This study shows that the outcomes of patients with erythema of rosacea and a high DMD treated with ivermectin 1% cream alone or combined with oral carvedilol showed a significantly reduced DMD, and their erythema was substantially improved. After 2018, we further noticed that the final DMD is very crucial, and patients are becoming more used to paying for drug treatment at their own expense, as well as that the efficacy of rosacea treatment has also been significantly improved.

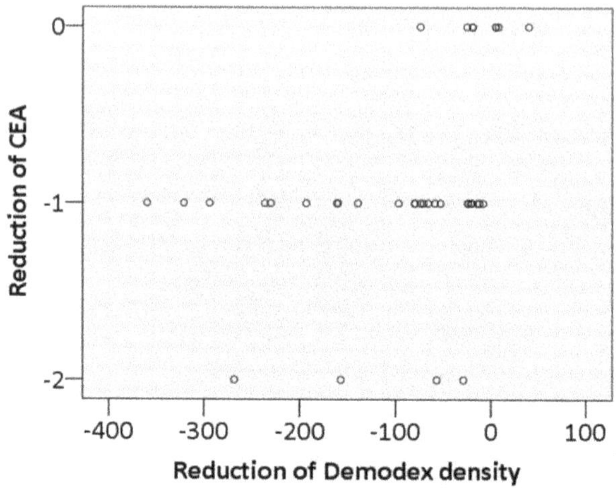


**Figure 54.** There is a significant correlation between the Clinician's Erythema Assessment and post-treatment reduction in *Demodex* density (Spearman's rho = 0.50, $p = 0.002$, n = 36). Reference: *Dermatol Ther.* 2021; 34(2): e14899.

## 2.10 Early exacerbation of rosacea induced by topical ivermectin treatment

Among the 39 patients mentioned in Section 2.9, five (12.8%) had local erythema and/or papulopustular exacerbation after treatment. These five cases were all patients with PPR, among whom four received ivermectin 1% cream only (23.5%) and one received combined treatment with carvedilol (4.5%). At the time, the effect of carvedilol on the incidence of exacerbation could not be explained until 2021 when J Zhang's research team found that carvedilol inhibits macrophage TLR-2 expression, thereby reducing the secretion of KLK-5 and the expression of LL-37, ultimately inhibiting the inflammatory response of rosacea.[11] This can clearly explain the lower incidence of exacerbation in the group treated with topical ivermectin combined with oral carvedilol than that in the group treated with ivermectin alone.

Exacerbation occurred on days 1–4 after starting ivermectin treatment, with one mild, two moderate, and three severe cases of reactions. One of the cases did not receive treatment, and the exacerbations resolved in the other four cases after 2 days to 2 weeks of treatment with topical or low-dose oral steroids. Two of the four patients continued to receive ivermectin 1% cream treatment, and one had an excellent outcome and the other had a good outcome (Table 7). Pustule biopsy of a patient with exacerbation was performed, and histopathology showed a superficial follicular pustule containing neutrophils and infiltration of lymphocytes around superficial blood vessels and hair follicles (Figures 55, 56). The

**Table 7.** Ivermectin cream for the treatment of exacerbating papulopustular and/or facial erythema caused by rosacea

| | IVM (n = 17) | IVM-CAR (n = 22) | Total (n = 39) |
|---|---|---|---|
| ETR | 0 | 0 | 0 |
| PPR | 4 | 1 | 5 |
| Total | 4 (24%) | 1 (4.5%) | 5 (12.8%) |

Note: IVM, ivermectin 1% cream; IVM-CAR, ivermectin 1% cream combined with carvedilol; ETR, Erythematotelangiectatic rosacea; PPR, Papulopustular rosacea

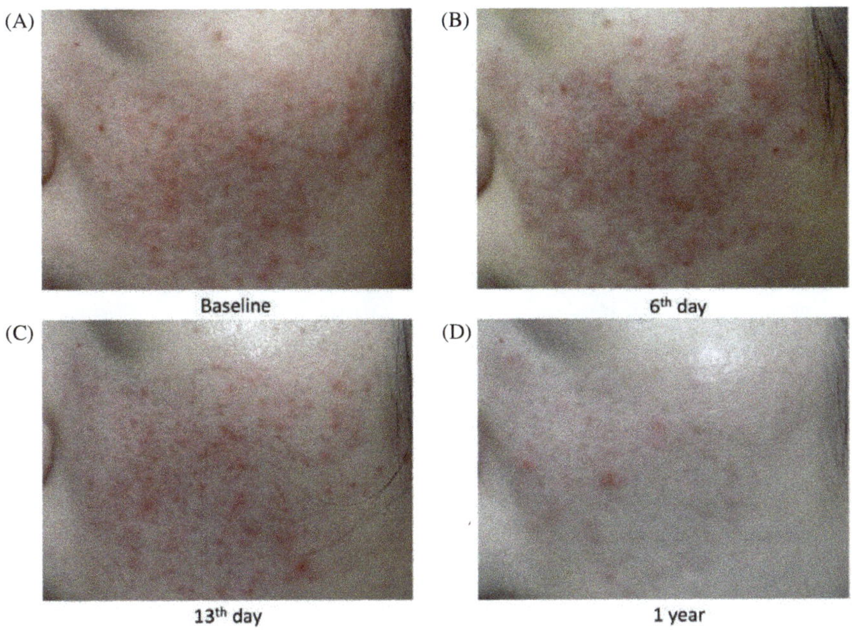


**Figure 55.** A female patient with rosacea before treatment with ivermectin cream (A), two days after the exacerbation of papulopustular and erythematous lesions (B). Exacerbation subsided after treatment with steroids (C). Subsequently, the patient returned to the clinic after one year (D). Her *Demodex* density was 100 mites/cm$^2$ before treatment, with 26 mites/cm$^2$ remaining on the sixth day, 4 mites/cm$^2$ remaining on the 13th day, and 40 mites/cm$^2$ after 1 year. References: *Dermatol Ther*. 2021;34(2):e14899.

(A) (B) (C)

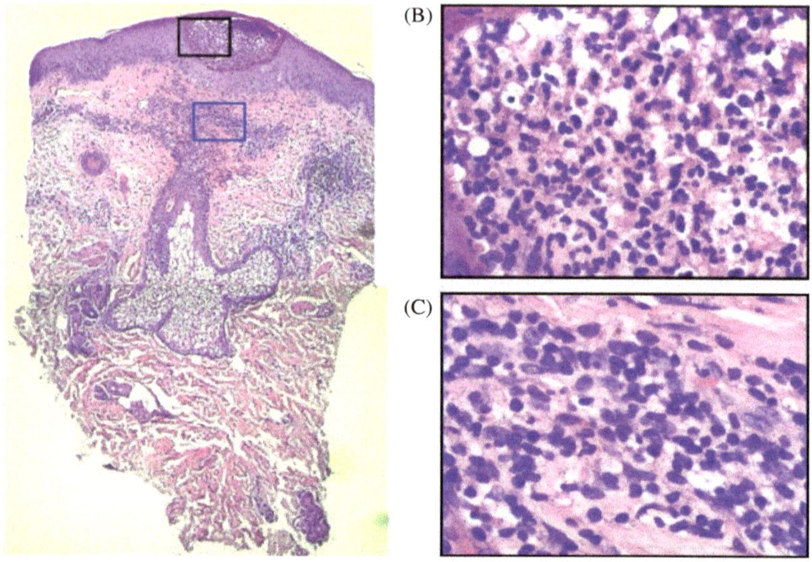

**Figure 56.** Histopathology of the case in Figure 55. There are a superficial follicular pustule and inflammatory cell infiltration around the superficial blood vessels and around the hair follicle in the dermis (A), The pustule contains neutrophils (B). Infiltrating cells around blood vessels are small lymphocytes and histiocytes (C). H&E stain, original magnification (A) 40x, (B, C) 400x.

exacerbation disappeared after treatment with steroids. The DMD before treatment was 100 mites/cm$^2$. On the sixth day, 26 mites/cm$^2$ remained, and on the 13th day, 4 mites/cm$^2$ remained, showing a worsening reaction accompanied by the death of a large number of *Demodex* mites (Figures 55, 56). Four patients with increased DMD took oral isotretinoin at 10–20 mg/day for 6–7 weeks. The DMD reduced to 0–10 mites/cm$^2$, and one patient needed additional metronidazole gel 0.75% to help control *Demodex* mites.

Topical ivermectin has been reported to improve erythema in patients with mild ETR, but the report did not evaluate the DMD.[12] The efficacy of topical ivermectin in reducing erythema of rosacea may be achieved through anti-inflammatory response and by killing *Demodex* mites. Dead mites are an important initiating factor for Toll-like receptors. In this study, we found that topical ivermectin only or topical ivermectin combined with carvedilol resulted in significant improvement in erythema of rosacea and reduction in DMD. Carvedilol can effectively improve rosacea and flushing, acting quickly and allowing a gradual decrease in drug use. In some of our patients, carvedilol effectively reduced the local exacerbation reaction caused by topical ivermectin and allowed a faster and earlier control of rosacea.

## 2.11 Mechanism of rosacea exacerbation at the early stage in topical ivermectin treatment and prevention methods

Topical ivermectin treatment at the early stage may exacerbate rosacea. This exacerbation can be treated with steroids. Thus, what is the mechanism of exacerbation? Is it possible to use topical steroids in the initial treatment stage to prevent and terminate such adverse reactions in the early stage?

In this series of studies, we first enrolled 23 patients, including 17 patients with rosacea and 6 patients with demodicosis, and administered five small pea-sized doses of approximately 0.3 g of topical ivermectin cream twice a day. The TSM was used to detect mites; DMD was recorded weekly to obtain the reduction ratio curve of *Demodex* mites, with an average reduction of 75% in the first week (n = 3), 68% in the second week (n = 15), and 78% in the third week (n = 9).

We also found that the antiparasitic effect of topical ivermectin is related to the dosage (Figure 57). Application of the following dosages showed that the antiparasitic effect increases gradually: an amount of five small pea sizes twice a day, an amount of two index finger tip units once a day, and an amount of two index finger tip units twice a day. The amount of two index finger tip units is equivalent to 1 g. The average 2-week reduction rate of mites is 67% for the amount of five small peas used twice a day, 84% for two index finger tip units at night, and 98.5% for two index finger tip units twice a day (Figure 58). Although different doses of topical ivermectin have varying degrees of antiparasitic effect, the highest number of *Demodex* mites die within the first week.

In 2017 and 2018, we investigated the application of different dosages of topical ivermectin: five pea-sized amount every morning and evening, an amount of two index finger tip units every night, 0.3 g every morning and evening, and an amount of two index finger tip units each morning

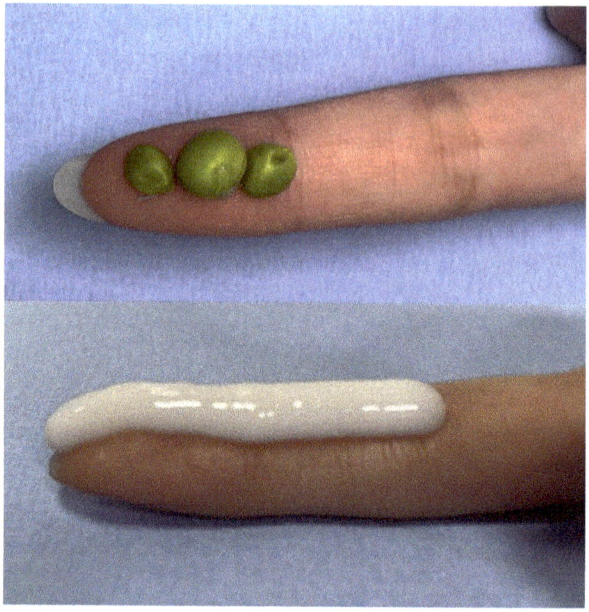

**Figure 57.** The amount of the drug is measured in terms of the number of peas in the picture above. The size of peas varies substantially. The amount in two index finger tip units in the figure below is about 1g.

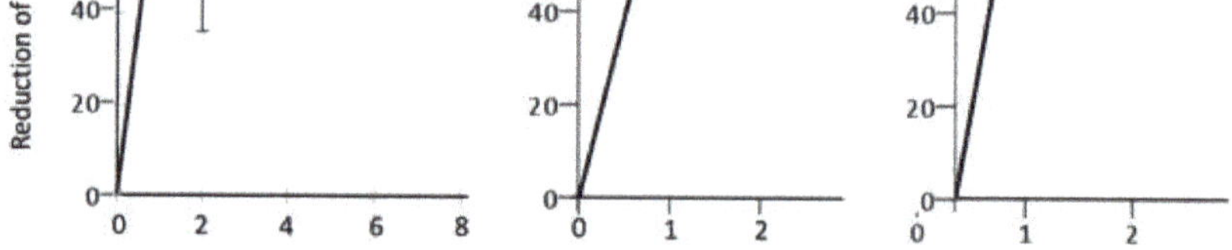


**Figure 58.** Comparison of the application of topical ivermectin of the following dosages: an amount of five small peas (approximately 0.3 g) twice a day, an amount of two index finger tip units once a day (approximately 1 g), and an amount of two index finger tip units twice a day (approximately 2 g). The antiparasitic effect increases gradually, with the average 2-week mite reduction rate being 67%, 84%, and 98.5%, respectively.

and evening, with the TSM for sampling to observe the pattern of mites under the microscope at regular intervals. The sampling times were 8, 12, and 24 hours, as well as on the 2nd, 3rd, 4th, 5th, 6th, 7th, and 14th days of application. The results showed that dead mites could only be found 12 h after the application of all three dosages. Small-sized mites were dead in those receiving five pea-sized-amount in the morning and at night, whereas medium- and large-sized mites were not affected. Those receiving 1 g per night were found with medium-sized mites dead, and those receiving 1 g each in the morning and at night were found with many large-, medium-, and small-sized mites dead (Figure 59). In the first week, a group of dead mites could be observed in a lump of sebum (Figures 60 and 61). After a week, only sporadic distribution of dead mites was observed, and sometimes, there were no traces of dead mites.

We also performed a blue filter examination under a fluorescence microscope. In three patients with rosacea, the DMD before treatment was $247 \pm 116$ mites/cm$^2$. They were treated with 1 g of topical ivermectin for

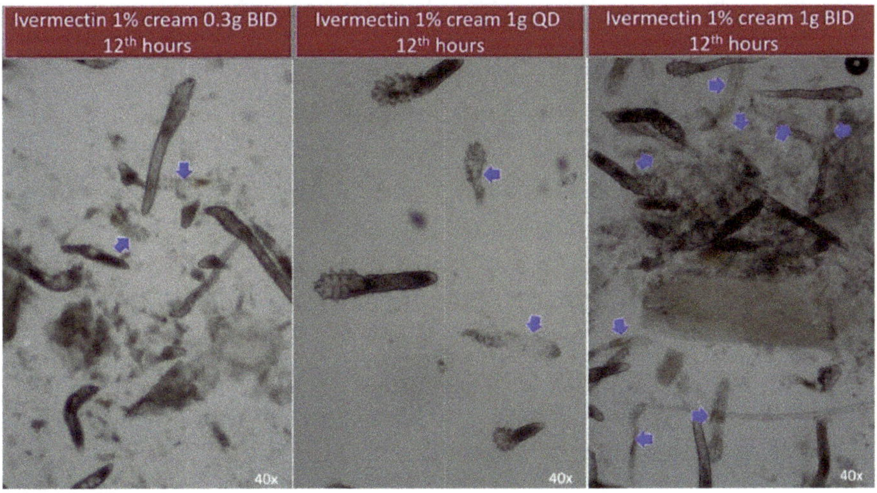


**Figure 59.** Based on the antiparasitic effects of ivermectin 1% cream on *Demodex* mites, it requires >12 h for the treatment of either of the three dosages to see dead mites. The death of small-sized mites was observed with the treatment of 0.3 g in the morning and at night, where medium- and large-sized mites were not affected. In contrast, those receiving 1 g per night were found with medium-sized mites dead, and those receiving 1 g each in the morning and at night were found with many large-, medium-, and small-sized mites dead.

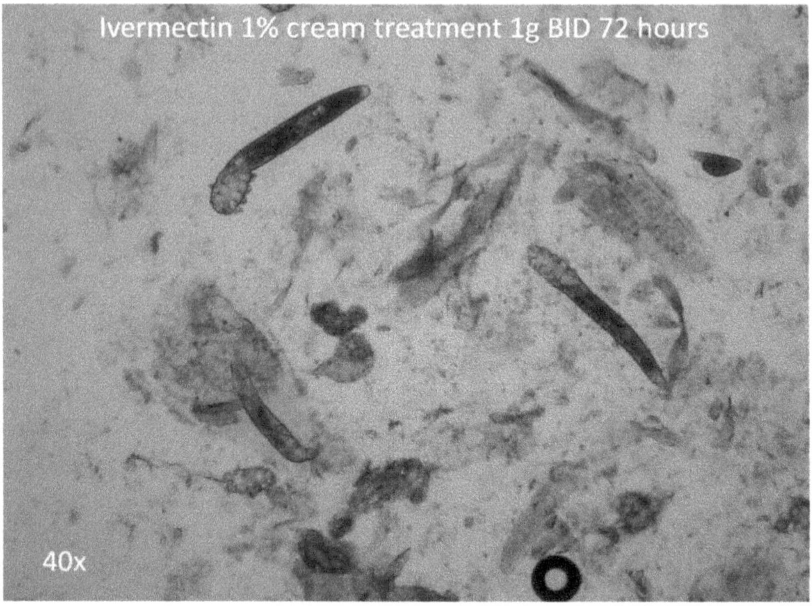


**Figure 60.** Ivermectin 1% cream treatment (1-g BID for 72 h) caused the death of many large-sized mites.

7 days and were sampled using the TSM. In these samples, the alive mites were active, with their exoskeleton, claws, and main parts of the internal organs showing spontaneous emission of blue fluorescence. Those mites that were dead lost their mobility with the whole body showing spontaneous emission. Under the microscope, clusters of dead mites could be found at many sites (Figure 61). Five samples were collected from three patients. The ratio of dead to alive adult mites at the time of one week was 0.08–0.91, and the mean ± standard deviation was 0.45 ± 0.34. The results showed that at the time of one week of treatment, some patients had many dead mites remaining in their hair follicles.

Based on the findings, about 70%–80% of the mites died in the first week, and many groups of dead mites were found under the fluorescence microscope in the same hair follicle (Figure 62). This coincided with the time of the exacerbation of rosacea in patients receiving ivermectin cream in their early stage of treatment, which was mentioned earlier in Section 2.10.

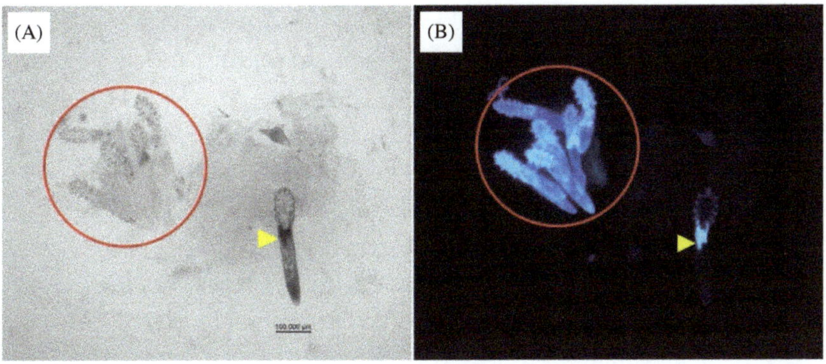


**Figure 61.** Antiparasitic effect of ivermectin 1% cream on *Demodex* mites showed, via the TSM, adult mites alive with good mobility and complete body shape under an ordinary optical microscope (A, yellow arrow), dead adult mites were immobile and disintegrated (A, red circles). Under the fluorescence microscope with a blue filter, those mites alive were active, with their exoskeleton, claws, and main internal organs showing spontaneous emission of blue fluorescence. Those mites dead lost their mobility, with the whole body showing spontaneous emission (B, yellow arrow). Clusters of dead mites could be found (B, red circles).

Reference: *Dermatol Ther*. 2022 Jul;35(7):e15517.

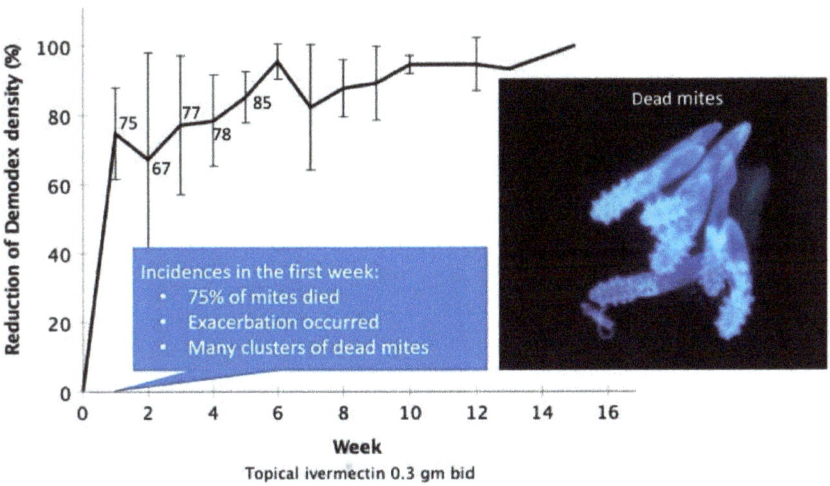


**Figure 62.** Antiparasitic effect of ivermectin 1% cream on *Demodex* mites showed, based on our studies, that ivermectin cream induces exacerbation of rosacea in the early treatment stage, which usually occurs in the first week. This is also the time when nearly 75% of the mites die, and many clusters of dead mites can be found under the fluorescence microscope.

Reference: *Dermatol Ther*. 2022 Jul;35(7):e15517.

The fourth part of the study included 178 patients with rosacea and high DMD. They received two finger tip units of topical ivermectin once at night. They were also given low-potency steroids for preventive purposes. Patients were instructed to apply topical steroids immediately once new papules and pustules or local erythema occurred. Usually, steroids were no longer needed after a week. After excluding 30 cases with whom we lost contact during follow-up, two of the remaining 146 cases (1.4%) developed obvious pustular exacerbation on the fifth day and required treatment. After detailed questioning, it turned out that the patients read too much online information and were afraid of using steroids. They missed their treatment opportunity when the first pustules appeared, and subsequently, dozens of papules and pustules appeared the next day. The exacerbation rate of this treatment was much lower than that of another treatment of 12.8% in the study on 39 patients that we previously mentioned.

From our studies, we found that ivermectin cream induces exacerbation of rosacea in the early treatment stage, which usually occurs in the first week. This is also the time when nearly 75% of the mites die, and many clusters of dead mites can be found under the fluorescence microscope. In the same hair follicle, the chitin in dead mites' exoskeleton and the bacteria and metabolic waste in the body will dissolve. Chitin is known to induce the expression of Toll-like receptors in keratinocytes, thereby causing innate immune responses.[13] Bacteria and metabolic waste in the body can cause immune cell differentiation and leukocyte chemotactic response.[14,15] These innate and acquired immune responses can be prevented and treated through the early use of low-potency topical steroids (Figure 63). This research was jointly published by Prof. Lee Yu-Yun, Prof. Hsu Chao-Kai, and Dr. Huang Hui-Peng in Dermatol Ther. 2022;35(7):e15517.[16]

## 2.12 *Demodex* resistance to topical ivermectin

*Demodex* mites treated with topical ivermectin may not decrease as expected or even increase because the medicine used is too little, the medicine is not used on time, or that the mites are resistant to the medicine. We had a case of a young woman who had been using oral isotretinoin for a long time to treat PPR. Every time she stopped the isotretinoin, she faced the relapse of

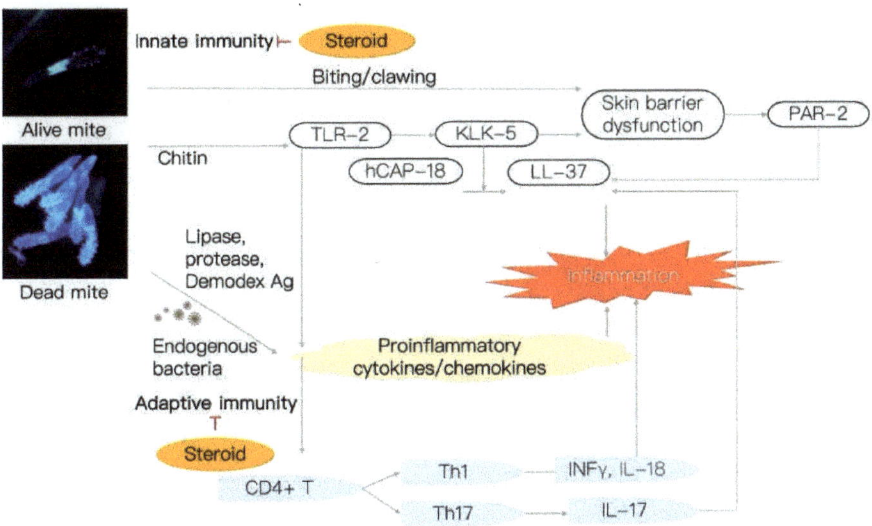


**Figure 63.** Ivermectin 1% cream may cause early exacerbation of the disease. In the presence of clusters of dead mites in a follicle, the chitin in the dead mites' exoskeleton and the bacteria and metabolic waste in the body degrade. Chitin is known to induce the expression of Toll-like receptors in keratinocytes, thereby causing innate immune responses. Bacteria and metabolic waste in the body can cause immune cell differentiation and leukocyte chemotactic response. These innate and acquired immune responses can be prevented and treated through the early use of low-potency topical steroids.

papulopustules. During the treatment of this patient, we tested the density of *Demodex* mites on her face, which was 41 mites/cm$^2$; thus, topical ivermectin treatment was administered. After 3 weeks, her papulopustules reduced, and the mite density dropped to 31 mites/cm$^2$. However, during the fifth week, her papulopustules and DMD increased. During the seventh week of treatment, oral isotretinoin was added to her treatment again.

The dosage of oral isotretinoin was 20 g daily. In the 12th week, her papulopustules were completely gone, and her DMD was 0 mites/cm$^2$. After 6 months of continuous treatment, the dosage of oral isotretinoin was finally reduced to 10 mg every 5 days (Figure 64). The 3-year follow-up via phone revealed that the patient had stopped taking medication and remained asymptomatic.

Oral isotretinoin inhibits the secretion of sebaceous glands. We found in another clinical case of ours that after regular mite inspection, the body

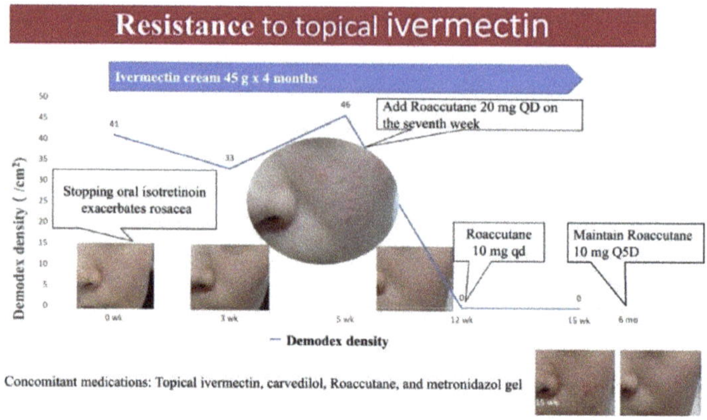


**Figure 64.** *Demodex* mites may increase during topical ivermectin treatment. A young woman with PPR was treated with oral isotretinoin for a long time. The papulopustules recurred every time the medicine was stopped. The density of *Demodex* mites tested by the TSM was 41 mites/cm$^2$, so she started treatment with topical ivermectin. After 3 weeks, the papulopustules reduced, and the mite density dropped to 31 mites/cm$^2$. However, the papulopustules deteriorated and mite density increased during the fifth week. During the seventh week, the patient reintroduced isotretinoin 20 mg daily. During the 12th week of the follow-up visit, she showed no papulopustules or detection of mites. After 6 months of continuous treatment, the oral retinoic acid dose could finally be reduced to 10 mg every 5 days.

size of *Demodex* mites did not change after treatment with 30 g of topical ivermectin and 30 g of topical permethrin. In contrast, with the treatment of oral isotretinoin at 10 mg/day for 3 weeks, the size of the *Demodex* mites became smaller, with body length reduced by 29% (Figure 65). We also found smaller-than-average *Demodex* mites in four other patients who received isotretinoin treatment. The doses that these patients received were 10 mg/day for 4 weeks, 10 mg/day for 10 weeks, 20 mg/day for 10 weeks, and 20 mg/3 days for 4 months. Sebum, the nutritional source of the mite larvae, is considered to be inhibited and reduced, resulting in the maldevelopment of mites. Therefore, in clinical practice, we often use oral isotretinoin combined with topical ivermectin to treat patients whose *Demodex* mites reduce less quickly than expected. Topical permethrin and topical metronidazole can also be useful for some patients whose mites show resistance to topical ivermectin treatment.

There was also a patient whose DMD dropped from 500 mites/cm$^2$ to 119 mites/cm$^2$. Subsequently, we could not further reduce the mites.

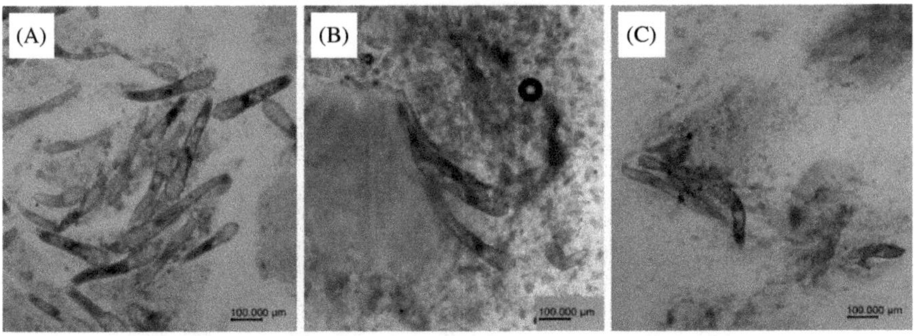


**Figure 65.** Effects of oral isotretinoin on *Demodex* mites. (A) Before treatment, the *Demodex* mite density was 574 mites/cm$^2$ (B). After 7 weeks of treatment with topical ivermectin 30 g and topical permethrin 30 g, only large mites remained, whereas small-sized ones were cleared up. The density of mites was 7 *D. folliculorum* + 12 *D. brevis*/cm$^2$ (C). With the treatment of isotretinoin 10 mg daily for 3 weeks, mites became smaller, and their body length reduced by 29%.

Fortunately, so far, we have not seen any case whose demodicosis was effectively treated with topical ivermectin yet turned into resistant.

## 2.13 Are there seasonal differences in demodicosis?

Data from Huang Hui-Peng Dermatological Clinic from January 2019 to December 2021 on patients who received topical ivermectin, where only their first visit was considered, showed no seasonal differences in demodicosis. However, more patients visited the clinic in January and July. In summer, under the influence of heat waves and rainfall, more patients are expected to seek medical help (Figure 66).

## 2.14 Are small pustules after laser treatments related to *Demodex*?

Some patients develop small pustules after Q-switch laser toning and picosecond laser treatment. Examination of the pustules with the superficial needle-scraping method showed that some of them contained *Demodex* mites that exceeded the diagnostic criteria (Figure 67), and some of them contained mites in a normal range (Figure 68). Therefore, before receiving full-face laser treatment, people should first get screened for excessive DMD. In cases where DMD is too high, it is safer to use

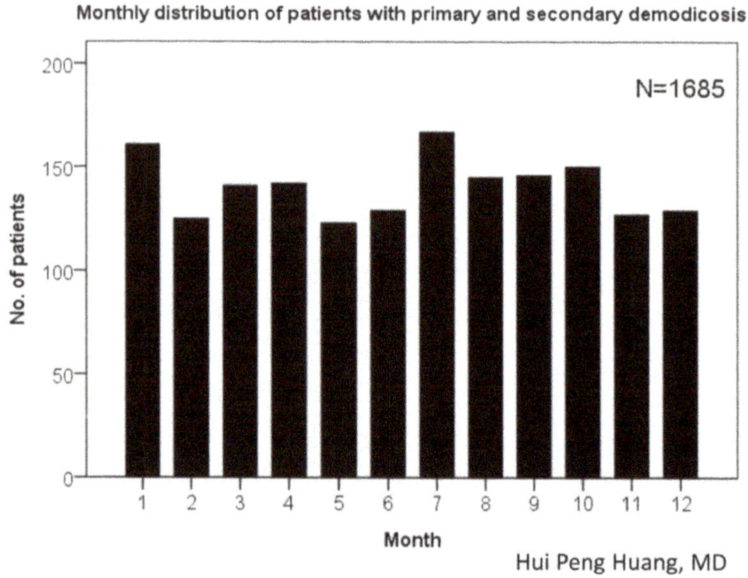


**Figure 66.** Monthly distribution of 1,685 cases receiving topical ivermectin over 3 years showed no significant seasonal differences but there were slightly more patients in January and July.

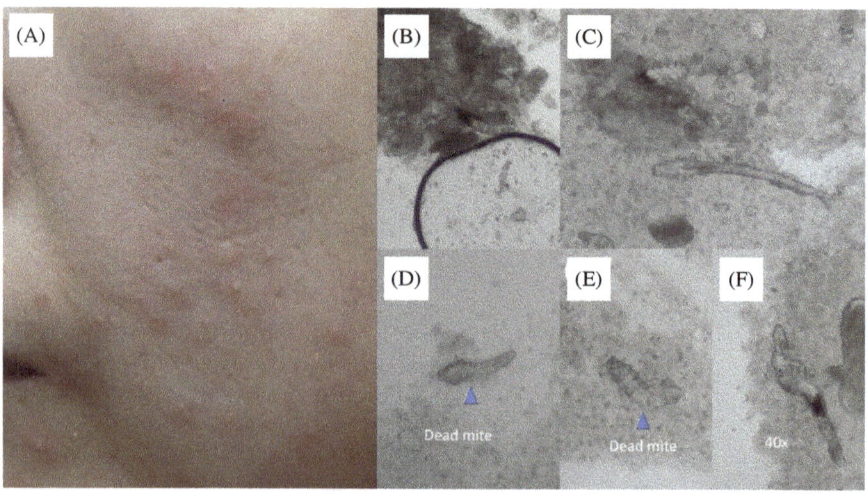


**Figure 67.** After the patient received picosecond laser treatment, small pustules appeared the next day. The pustules were examined using the superficial needle-scraping method. Six *Demodex* mites were found from five pustules, and two mites were dead. The laser might kill the mites, which in turn causes an inflammatory reaction.

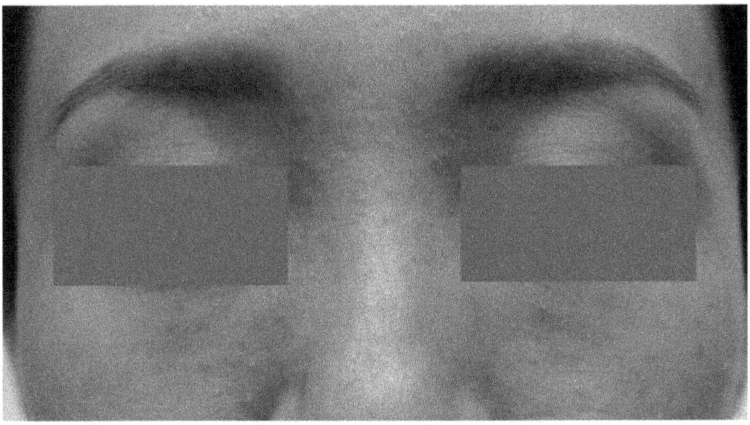

**Figure 68.** After the patient received Nd:YAG laser treatment twice, small pustules appeared the next day. Superficial needle-scraping for pustules showed no *Demodex* mites in five pustules. It could be irritant folliculitis caused by the laser.

topical ivermectin to reduce the number of mites before undergoing laser treatment. As a precaution to *Demodex*-related pustules after laser surgery, low-potency topical steroids can be prescribed first, and topical ivermectin can be prescribed simultaneously.

## 2.15 Ocular demodicosis

In the past, when dermatologists studied ocular rosacea and ocular demodicosis, they often found this topic hard to understand and even chose to skip it. In 2019, we decided to delve into this challenging topic and presented case reports of 18 cases with ocular demodicosis at a meeting by the Taiwanese Dermatology Association. In ocular rosacea, *Demodex folliculorum* mites infest the eyelash follicles, and *Demodex brevis* mites infest the meibomian glands. Manifestations of ocular *Demodex* infection reported in studies include pathognomonic cylindrical dandruff and noncharacteristic greasy scales.[17] Cylindrical dandruff refers to lesions located on the eyelashes, characterized by scabs covering the roots in columnar shape. Itching is the most prominent symptom associated with ocular demodicosis.[18] In a review study of 844 patients with papulopustules and demodicosis, 21% had eye involvement, and 18% were found with *Demodex* mites on their eyelids.[19] In our report,

18 patients with ocular demodicosis were included. The patients included nine males and nine females, aged 29–64 years, and a child aged 1 year and 9 months, with an average age of 47.7 ± 11.8 years. Among them, 14 had rosacea on the face, 5 had ETR, 9 had PPR, 3 had seborrheic dermatitis, 2 had steroid-induced dermatitis, 1 had pityriasis folliculorum, and 2 had normal skin condition on the face. The test method was epilation of eyelashes. The clinical manifestations of ocular demodicosis in 11 cases were anterior blepharitis, including 10 cases of honey-like scale crust (Figure 69) and 1 case of eyelid margin erythema; 12 cases had styes (Figure 70), and the test results of the extracted eyelashes showed 1–28 *Demodex* mites detected in four eyelashes. There was one case involving the collection of two *Demodex brevis* mites collected from a single sty. Based on the outcome, we found that topical ivermectin and a cleansing solution containing tea tree oil are efficacious for anterior blepharitis, where *Demodex* mites were cleared up after 1–2 weeks of treatment. In contrast, patients with styes require a longer treatment duration, usually more than a month, and hot compress and massage are usually required.

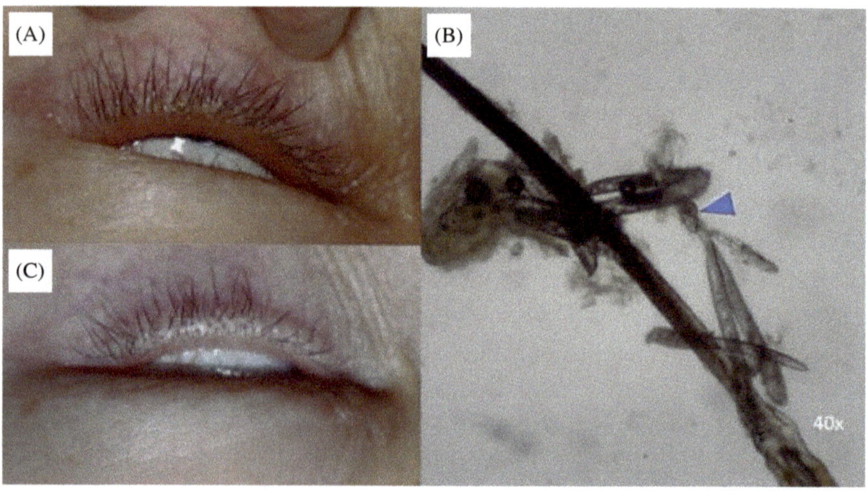


**Figure 69.** Demodicosis of the eyes. (A) honey-like scale crust in anterior blepharitis; (B) one eyelash sample for examination revealed 12 mites and a total of 16 mites in four eyelash samples. The blue arrow indicates an egg. (C) After one week of treatment with topical ivermectin, the honey-like scale crust disappeared and no *Demodex* mites were detected.

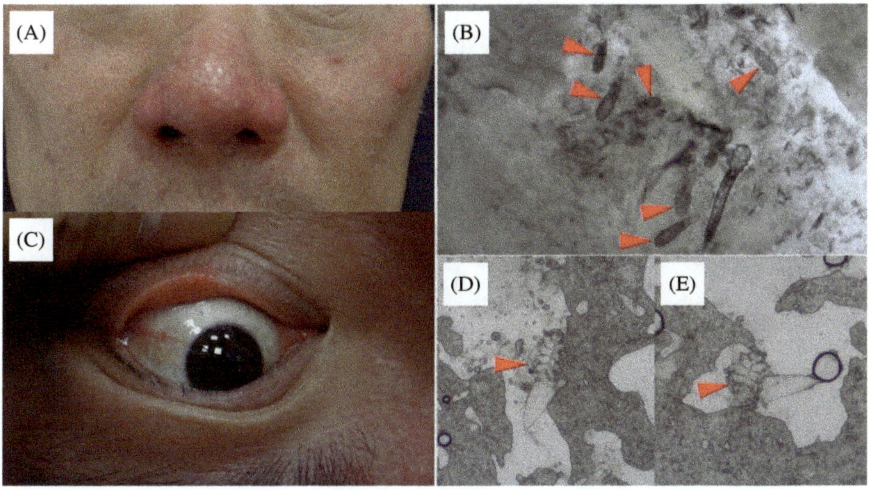


**Figure 70.** Ocular demodicosis. (A) A male patient with rosacea (B), whose thumbnail-squeezing test revealed 171 *Demodex* mites/cm$^2$, most of which were *Demodex brevis* (red arrow); (C) a sty at the left lower eyelid; (D, E) the thumbnail-squeezing test showed two *Demodex brevis* mites in the meibomian glands (red arrow), featured by the cone-like tails.

Among the 12 patients with styes, 3 had a high density of *Demodex* mites on their faces, and 1 was a child who had a recurrent sty.

The method of applying topical ivermectin to the eyelids is as follows: use a small cotton swab to take a dose the size of two sesame seeds at a time and apply it to the lowest edge of the lower eyelashes (Figure 71), once a day before going to bed. Subsequently, wash the eyelashes immediately after waking up. No medication is required on the upper eyelids because they come in contact with the lower eyelids when the eyes are closed while sleeping. Notably, patients who lose their eyelashes in the lower eyelids may find this method of application irritating to their eyes.

What role should the dermatologist play in ocular demodicosis? I think they should be capable of diagnosing ocular demodicosis in patients with rosacea. Cylindrical dandruff is a characteristic sign of ocular demodicosis (Figure 72). Noncharacteristic greasy scale crust and styes should be highly suspected. Itchy eyes and dry eyes are also important symptoms. The main test method is to take eyelash samples for examination. Before collecting eyelash samples, they can be touched lightly. Because of the shocks, mites may cling to the hair root tightly. To get a

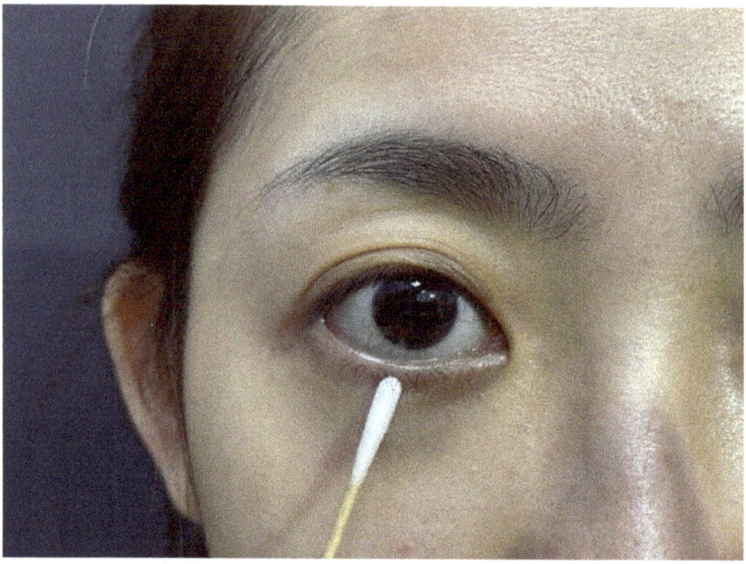

**Figure 71.** To apply topical ivermectin to the eyelids, use a small cotton swab to take a dose the size of two sesame seeds at a time and apply it to the lowest edge of the lower eyelashes once a day before going to bed. The eyelashes should be washed immediately after waking up. No medication is required on the upper eyelids because the upper eyelids come in contact with the lower eye lashes when the eyes are closed while sleeping.

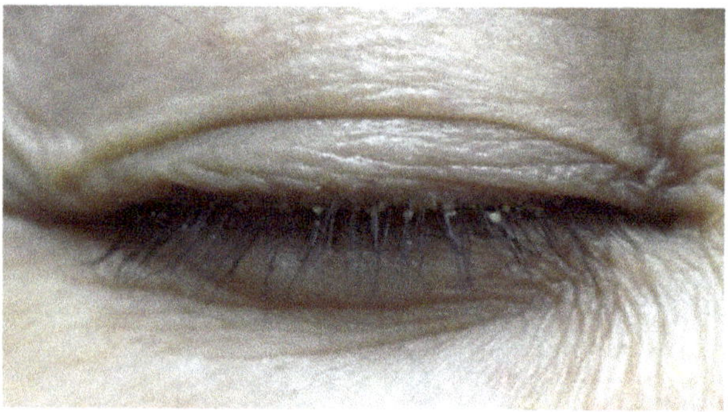

**Figure 72.** Cylindrical dandruff in a case of ocular demodicosis.

sample with mites on it, the sampling movement should be practiced slowly, sometimes even with a pause. Quick sampling is considered inappropriate. In addition to medical treatment and hot compress massages, cleaning the eyes is also important. Patients can use a small amount of shampoo to make a foam to clean their eyelids, followed by rinsing with clean water.

## 2.16 Is *Demodex* visible under a dermoscope?

Background: In 2010, Dr. Segal et al. first published the use of polarized dermoscopy as a tool for diagnosing demodicosis. They reported that 72 patients with facial rashes underwent clinical, microscopic, and dermoscopic examinations, and 55 of them were found with demodicosis. Dermoscopy showed 54 patients having *Demodex* tails and *Demodex* follicular openings. Microscopic examination of scraped skin tissue revealed *Demodex* mites in 52 cases, and they concluded that dermoscopy results were consistent with microscopy results (kappa value: 0.86, 95% CI: 0.72–0.99; $P < 0.001$).[20] The authors mentioned that there are three types of dermoscopic characteristics for demodicosis: *Demodex* tails, *Demodex* follicular openings and follicular scales, and full-sized *Demodex* mites (Figure 73).[20] Dr. Friedman et al. also reported a case of demodicosis whose dermoscopy result showed two characteristics: *Demodex* tails and *Demodex* follicular openings (Figure 74).[21]

To the best of my knowledge, the diameter of the tail of *Demodex* mites is much smaller than the diameter of follicular pores; thus, I conducted the following study.

Purpose: To verify the reports on demodicosis published by Dr. Segal and Dr. Friedman and to examine the appropriateness of the skin photographs and their findings.

Methods: I used a dermoscope (Heine NC2) to observe skin samples collected from patients who were found with enlarged pores and follicular plugs and suspected to have demodicosis, followed by SSSB and the TSM for sample collection. Next, used the dermatoscope to observe the collected samples and took photographs of them. Subsequently, compared the photos, after adjusting the zoom levels, with those from Dr. Segal and Dr. Friedman.[20,21]

Result: From the images of the vellus hairs and *Demodex* mites collected by SSSB, we found that the diameter of the tail end of *Demodex folliculorum* mites is approximately the same as the diameter of hair (Figure 75). I compared the size of the *Demodex* mites collected via the

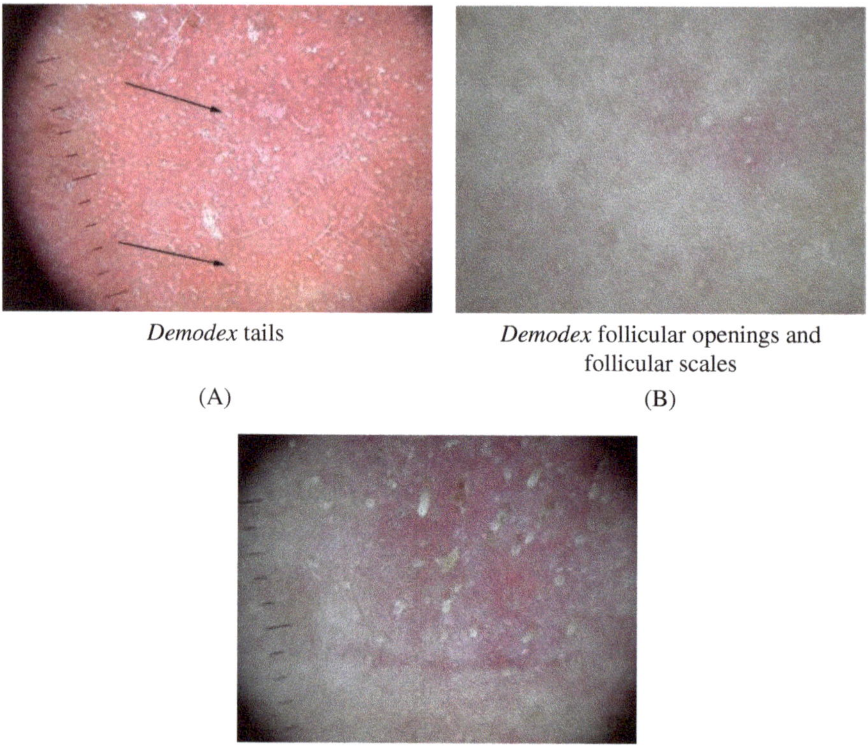

*Demodex* tails

(A)

*Demodex* follicular openings and follicular scales

(B)

Full-sized *Demodex* mite

(C)

**Figure 73.** Dr. Segal et al. published skin microscopic images of demodicosis, showing three types of findings: (A) *Demodex* tails, (B) *Demodex* follicular openings and follicular scales, and (C) full-sized *Demodex* mites.

Reference: *Int J Dermatol.* 2010 Sep; 49(9):1018–23.

TSM on the glass slide with that of follicular plugs in the images taken through a dermatoscope. Here, I found a ball of follicular plug in an enlarged follicle. Inside this ball of follicular plug, the white dot, whose diameter is the same as that of a vellus hair, is the tail end of a *Demodex* mite (Figure 76). The *Demodex* tails and full-sized *Demodex* mites described by Dr. Segal are significantly larger than the tails and bodies of *Demodex* mites sampled on glass slides (Figures 77 & 78).

Discussion: The magnification of a dermoscopy is only 6–10 times. Through dermoscopic observation, at most, enlarged pores, fine follicular

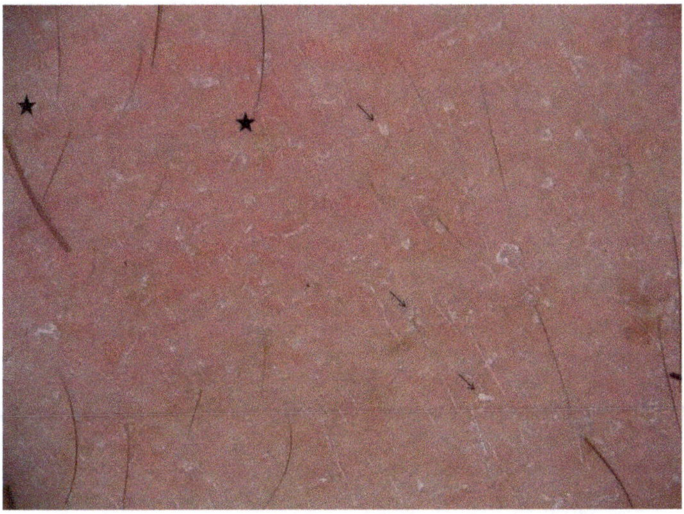

**Figure 74.** Dr. Friedman et al. published dermoscopic images of demodicosis, showing *Demodex* "tails" (arrow) and *Demodex* "follicular openings" (star).

Reference: Friedman et al. Usefulness of dermoscopy in the diagnosis and monitoring treatment of demodicidosis. *Dermatol Pract Concept*. 2017 Jan; 7(1):35–38.

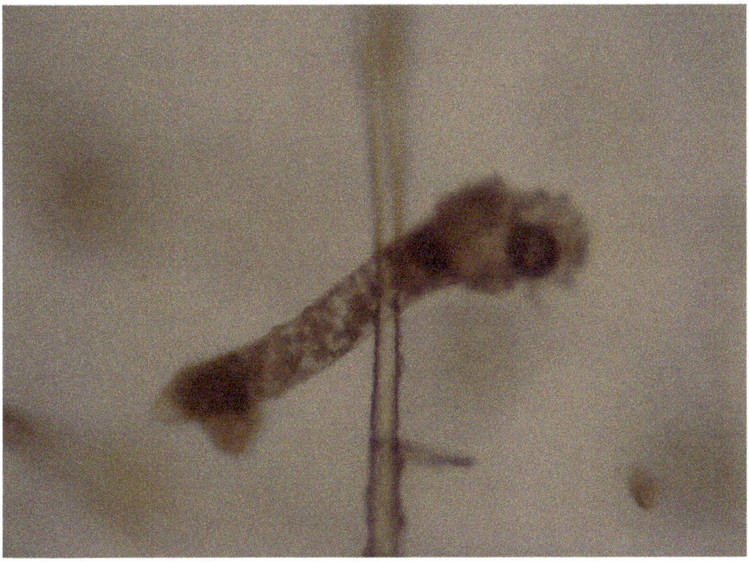

**Figure 75.** In the images of *Demodex* mites collected from the face using standardized skin surface biopsy, the diameter of the tail end of the mites is approximately the same as the diameter of the vellus hair.

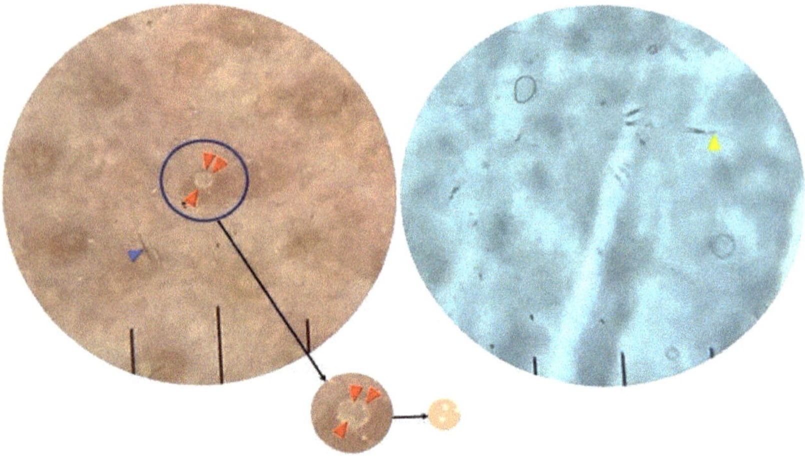

**Figure 76.** In the image on the left taken through a dermatoscope, there are many brown enlarged pores in the upper left part, and there are white plugs in the pores. In the white plug there are three smaller white spots (red arrows), whose diameters are similar to vellus hair (blue arrow) and as that of the tails (yellow arrow) of the *Demodex* mites on a glass slide shown in the image on the right. These fine white dots may be the tails of *Demodex* mites. The image below is a magnified picture of the white plug dot and their simulation.

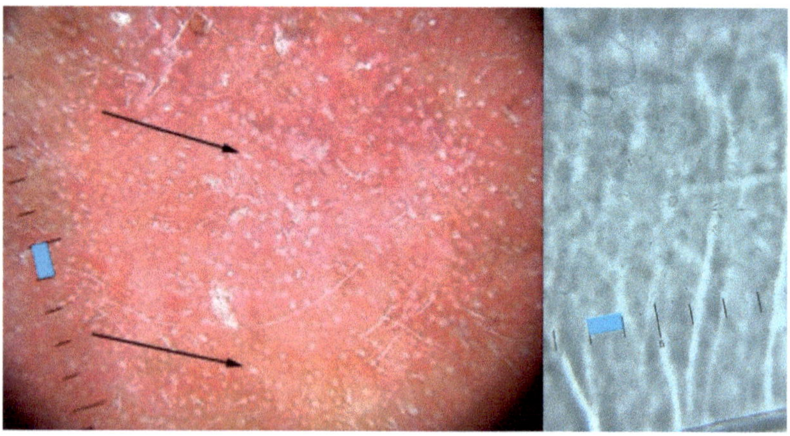

**Figure 77.** (Left) Rina Segal, MD, et al. Descriptions of *Demodex* tails. (Right) *Demodex folliculorum* collected by the TSM was smeared on a glass slide and photographed. After aligning, the actual size of the mite tail on the slide in the right picture was significantly smaller than the white dot in the left picture. Therefore, it is more reasonable that the Full-sized *Demodex* mite in the hair follicles described in the paper should be follicular plugs.

Reference: Dermoscopy as a diagnostic tool in demodicidosis. *Int J Dermatol*. 2010 Sep;49(9):1018–23.

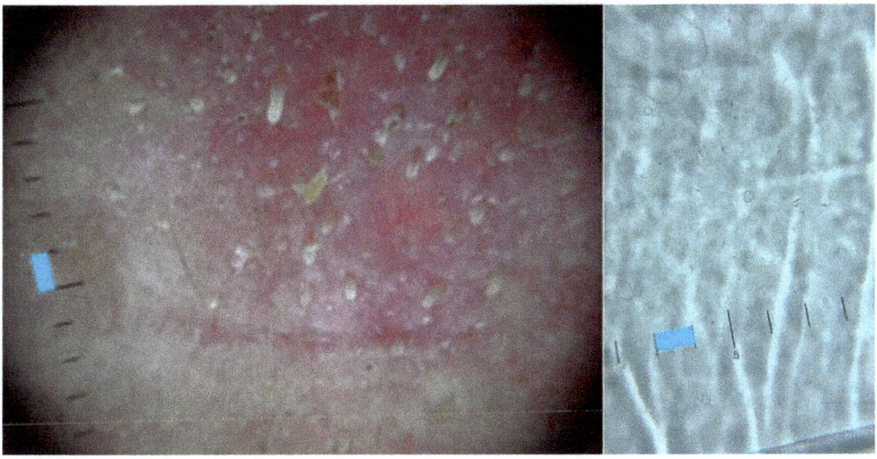

**Figure 78.** (Left) Rina Segal, MD, et al. The description of the full-sized *Demodex* mites migrating on the skin. (Right) *Demodex folliculorum* collected by the TSM was smeared on a glass slide and photographed. After aligning, the actual size of the mite on the slide in the right picture was significantly smaller than the white dot in the left picture. Therefore, it is more reasonable that the entire mites in the hair follicles described in the paper should be follicular scales.

Reference: Dermoscopy as a diagnostic tool in demodicidosis. *Int J Dermatol.* 2010 Sep;49(9): 1018–23.

plugs, or follicular scales can be seen. If the dermoscopy is connected to an iPhone to take photos for a zoomed-in view on a computer screen, even smaller white dots in the fine follicular plugs can be spotted. These white dots are the tail ends of *Demodex* mites, and it is fairly difficult to observe these dots using a dermatoscope alone. The dermatoscope images published by Dr. Segal and Dr. Friedman, considering *Demodex* mite infestation, are reasonable. However, the names they used to describe the patterns in the images may not be very accurate. The *Demodex* tail mentioned by Dr. Segal should be follicular scale, *Demodex* follicular opening and scales should be large pores with follicular plugs, and full-sized *Demodex* mites should be relatively large follicular scales (Table 8).

Moreover, these patterns are not exclusive to *Demodex* mite infestation and are commonly observed in conditions unrelated to *Demodex* mites. Similar symptoms have been reported in other inflammatory facial conditions such as acne, perioral dermatitis, tinea facies, rosacea, and

**Table 8.** A descriptive comparison of identical images of dermoscopic findings for demodicosis

| Segal et al. | Dr. Huang Hui-Peng |
|---|---|
| *Demodex* tails | Follicular scales |
| *Demodex* follicular openings and scales | Large hair pores and follicular plugs |
| Full-sized *Demodex* mite | Follicular scales |

seborrheic dermatitis.[22] I found similar dermoscopic images in my patients with sebaceous filaments, with only sebaceous substances but no *Demodex* mites (Figure 79).

Conclusion: It is not easy to spot the body of *Demodex* mites or their tails directly through a dermatoscope. Demodicosis should be considered when follicular scales and large pores with follicular plugs are seen under dermoscopy. Differential diagnosis for other diseases should also be considered.

## 2.17 Does *Demodex* cause large pores?

While discussing enlarged pores, experts often consider such pores in association with acne scars. If only the enlarged pores are considered, they can be mainly categorized by four major causes: mites, sebum, scars, and sagging skin.

1. An excessive increase in the number of *Demodex* mites can cause pores to burst. In the previous chapter, we discussed the nonpapulopustular type of demodicosis and its association with large pores. Enlarged pores may develop a coffee-colored or orange skin-like appearance or may become clogged with fine white contents inside the pore. This blockage is composed of a mixture of sebum, keratin, and *Demodex* mites (Figure 12).
2. Sebaceous hypersecretion causes sebum to accumulate into a solid sebaceous filament which enlarges the pore.
3. Post-acne fibrosis (acne scars).
4. Loose and sagging skin caused by decreased collagen makes pores appear enlarged.

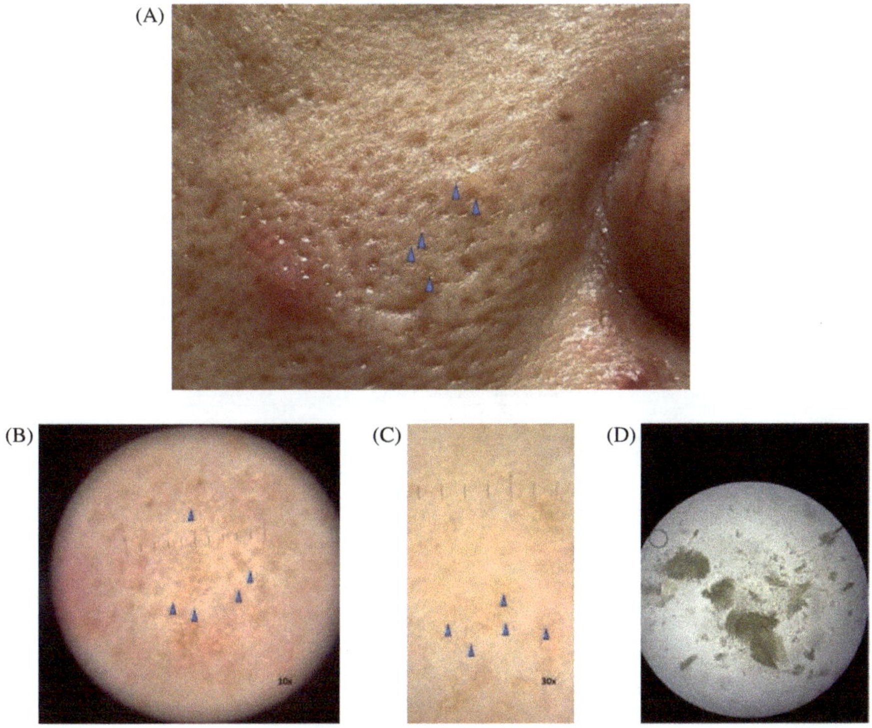

**Figure 79.** Sebaceous filament (A), Dermoscopic observation of white follicular plugs in enlarged pores, as the description of *Demodex* follicular openings and follicular scales by Segal et al. (indicated by blue arrows) (B, C). Samples taken using the thumbnail-squeezing method and viewed under the microscope showed only sebum, without mites (D).

The cause of large pores must be carefully identified, and the most appropriate method of treatment is selected in accordance with the cause to ensure that long-term results can be achieved. The TSM is a useful method for determining the causes of enlarged pores. The status of mites and solidified sebum within the hair follicle can be fairly assessed under a microscope (Figure 80). An excess of *Demodex* mites must be treated using an acaricide (Figure 81), and sebaceous hypersecretion must be treated using isotretinoin effectively. Other methods for controlling skin oiliness, such as skin peels, can improve keratinization by reducing the sebum and keratin remaining within the pores. Topical

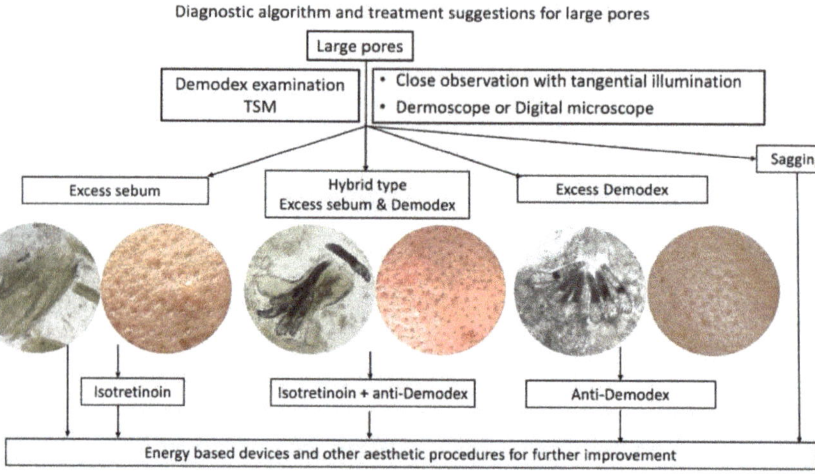


**Figure 80.** Diagnosis and treatment of enlarged pores. Scar is not included in the diagram.

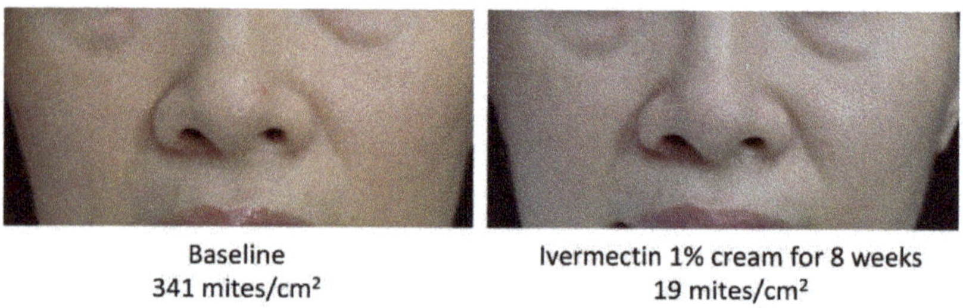


**Figure 81.** An excess of *Demodex* mites causes enlarged pores with an orange skin-like appearance. After treatment, the pores are visibly smaller and the skin is smoother.

oil-control skincare products are more often used to adsorb oil from the skin to prevent the oily face. Aging and sagging skin can be improved through a range of aesthetic medical devices and treatments. If the number of *Demodex* mites in a patient are not assessed, hasty use of lasers to shrink pores may result in post-treatment pustules and inflammation. These conditions are shown in Figures 68 and 69.

## 2.18 Retrospective evaluation of rosacea erythema treatment with pulsed dye lasers

Some previous research has claimed that pulsed dye lasers and intense pulsed light (IPL) can be used to treat ETR.[23–26] From November 2017 to November 2019, we retrospectively enrolled a total of 45 patients with rosacea, including 16 patients with PPR and 29 patients with ETR. We conducted a number of 118 treatments cumulatively. The patients were 22–73 years of age, with an average age of 44.7 ± 11.5 years, and had a history of rosacea ranging from 2 months to 30 years, with an average duration of 5.6 ± 7.4 years. All patients received two to ten treatments with a 585-nm pulsed dye laser, and the intervals between treatments ranged from 1 month to 1 year. Eight patients received additional 585-nm and 1064-nm dual wavelength (MultiPlex™) laser treatments, leading to 16 treatments cumulatively. The treatment parameters were as follows: 585 nm, 12 mm, 4 J/cm$^2$, 0.5 ms; MultiPlex™ 585 nm, 7 mm, 7–8 J/cm$^2$, 6 ms, 1064 mm, 60 J/cm$^2$, 10 ms, short delay (50–100 ms). Facial erythema was graded from 0 to 4 based on the five-point scale of the CEA, whereas papulopustules were graded from 0 to 4 based on the five-point scale of the Investigator's Global Assessment (IGA). We defined stable state rosacea as that which receives a grade ≤2 on the CEA scale or IGA scale and has a low DMD. We defined the treatment to be effective when facial erythema decreased and remained as such for >2 weeks, whereas treatment was deemed as having caused rosacea to flare-up when facial erythema increased and persisted for >2 days or in the event that more papulopustules occurred. All patients underwent a standard process of assessment and treatment (Figure 82). Some patients received prednisolone 5 mg t.i.d. after the pulsed dye laser treatment and were then monitored to assess whether post-laser treatment flare could be prevented.

Results: Of 118 treatments, 87 treatments had effective results (74%), whereas 4 treatments underwent symptom flare-up (3.4%). Of the 45 patients who received treatment, 34 patients had effective results (76%), whereas 3 patients experienced symptom flare-up induced by treatment (6.7%).

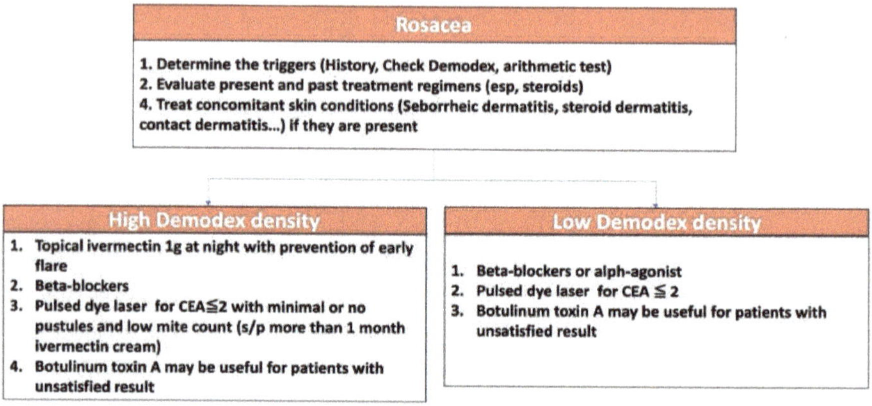


**Figure 82.** My standard procedure for the assessment and treatment of patients with rosacea using pulsed dye lasers. In cases with high *Demodex* density, new pustules may appear after pulsed dye laser treatment.

In terms of the total number of treatments, 84% of patients with stable state rosacea had effective treatment, whereas only half or 43% of patients with unstable state rosacea had effective treatment. Approximately 1.1% of stable state rosacea cases experienced post-treatment symptom flare-up, whereas 10% of unstable state rosacea cases experienced symptom flare-up, a number which is ten times higher (Figure 83, Table 9). There a patient who had previously obtained positive results from treatment experienced a sudden severe flare-up from the same treatment parameters, and the patient's skin could not return to its pretreatment condition by a year post-treatment.

Discussion: Pulsed dye lasers produce a visible wavelength of 585 nm or 595 nm and a pulse width of 0.45–40 ms. They exert a selective photothermal effect on red blood cells which absorb heat and transmit this heat to the capillaries causing coagulation or contraction, leading to collagen neogenesis in the dermis. According to the results of a study on the immunopathological responses of 32 patients undergoing pulsed dye laser treatment for rosacea, facial erythema was reduced in all patients after a single course of purpura-producing pulsed dye laser treatment, with a significant reduction in nerve fiber density and substance P immunoreactive nerve fibers. There was no significant difference between CGRP-positive nerve fibers and VIP-positive nerve fibers.[27] Thermal stimulation causes

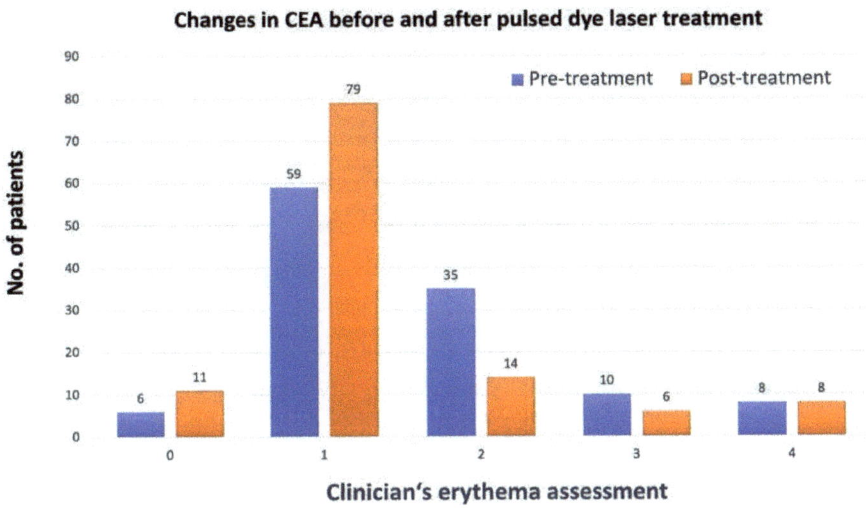


**Figure 83.** Changes in the Clinician's Erythema Assessment (CEA) grade of patients with rosacea before and after pulsed dye laser treatment. The blue bars represent pretreatment CEA grades, whereas the orange bars represent post-treatment CEA grades. There is an improvement in post-treatment erythema, as shown by an increase in patients with a CEA grade ≤1.

**Table 9.** Summary of pulsed dye laser treatment for rosacea

| Attributes | Session no. (n = 118) Effective/Flaring | Case no. (n = 45) Effective/Flaring |
|---|---|---|
| As a group | 87 (74%)/4 (3.4%) | 34 (76%)/3 (6.7%) |
| Stable state (n = 88) | 77 (84%)*/1 (1.1%)† | |
| Unstable state (n = 30) | 13 (43%)*/3 (10%)† | |
| Post-laser oral steroids‡ | | |
| No (n = 57) | 45 (79%)/3 (5%)§ | |
| Yes (n = 61) | 42 (69%)/1 (3%)§ | |

*, $p = 0.000$; †, $p = 0.020$; ‡, baseline erythema ($p = 0.020$); §, $p = 0.216$.

rosacea to flare-up, and thus the flare of erythema after pulsed dye laser treatment is probably related to thermal stimulation.

In conclusion, pulsed dye treatment is effective for the majority of patients with stable state rosacea (Figure 84). However, a minority of

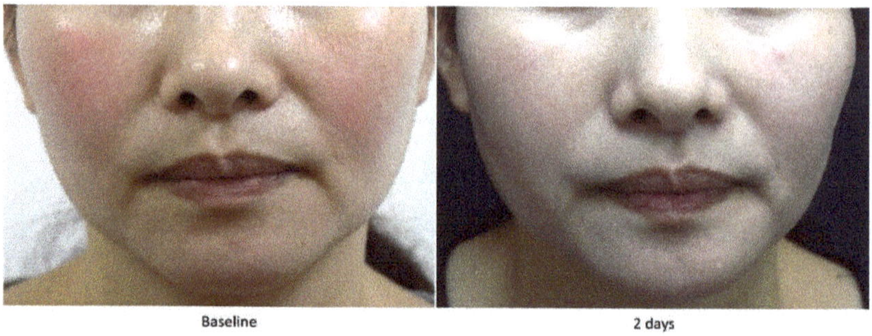


**Figure 84.** Comparison of a patient with rosacea before and two days after pulsed dye laser treatment. Erythema was markedly reduced.

patients will undergo post-treatment symptom flare, and their skin may even be unable to recover to its pretreatment condition. This is the major limitation of treatment with pulsed dye lasers.

## 2.19 Neurovascular response to rosacea caused by thermal stimulation and emotional stress

There are many pathogenic factors which may induce rosacea. One such factor is *Demodex*, which triggers an immune response, for which an effective treatment method has already been developed. The treatment allows for the effective control and alleviation of the rosacea, papulopustules, and erythema caused by *Demodex*.[7,10,16]

The primary pathways for neurovascular responses are thermal stimulation and emotional stress. In previous studies on rosacea, thermal stimulation has been described to primarily activate TRPV1, leading to the release of vasoactive peptides, which in turn causes vasodilation and the activation of downstream mast cells, macrophages, and neutrophils. This results in a subsequent inflammatory response.[28] However, in 1995, Kellogg studied cutaneous active vasodilation. The results indicated that according to the response mechanism, thermal stimulation can be divided into either whole body heating or local heating. Whole body heating activates the cholinergic branch of the sympathetic nervous system, which releases acetylcholine and cotransmitters dilates cutaneous arterioles. It has not yet been determined as to whether this cotransmitter is a VIP, and experiments have confirmed that acetylcholine plays only a small role in dilating cutaneous arterioles. Intradermal injection of botulinum toxin can inhibit the vasodilation response of the cholinergic branch of the sympathetic nervous system.[29] In 2017, Yamazaki noted that cutaneous vasodilation of the sympathetic nervous system also involves substances such as NO (neuronal nitric oxide synthase [nNOS]), substance P, VIP, PACAP, histamine, and prostaglandin.[30] We gave hydroxocobalamin which bound with NO to patients with rosacea and found that the flushing induced by the arithmetic test was substantially reduced in comparison with pretreatment levels. This indirectly confirms that NO is involved. When normal skin is heated locally to a temperature ≤42 °C, blood flow increases spontaneously, which in turn leads to a two-stage cutaneous vasodilation response (Figure 85). When skin is heated to ≥43 °C, this can act as a harmful irritant which causes nociceptive pain.

The initial increase in the blood flow to skin after non-nociceptive local heating is accompanied by a sensory nerve reflex, *viz*., the activation of the afferent C fibers, which cause vasodilation through the antidromic release of substance P and CGRP from sensory nerve endings. Additionally, the subsequent release of neuropeptide Y from adrenergic sympathetic nerve endings in the vicinity of the heated area of skin leads to a transient decrease in blood flow. Subsequently, the blood flow gradually increases to a stable plateau. This persistent vasodilation is associated with the generation of NO.[30–32] Another study on facial skin sympathetic activity found that the sympathetic nervous system activity in the skin of patients with rosacea under whole body heating and psychological or physiological stress is more active than that of normal people. In terms of increased blood flow caused by nociceptive localized thermal stimulation, the lesions were more visible on patients with PPR than normal people, but no significant different could be seen in patients with ETR.[33]

To summarize, we have plotted a graph (Figure 86) which represents the relationship between thermal stimulation, stress, sympathetic nervous system activity, sensory nerves, and NO. The graph illustrates the effects of thermal stimulation and psychological and physical stress on blood flow in the skin. Whole body heating and stress (physical or psychological) activate the sympathetic cholinergic nerve in the skin, which in turn causes vasodilation in the cutaneous arterioles. When thermal stimulation

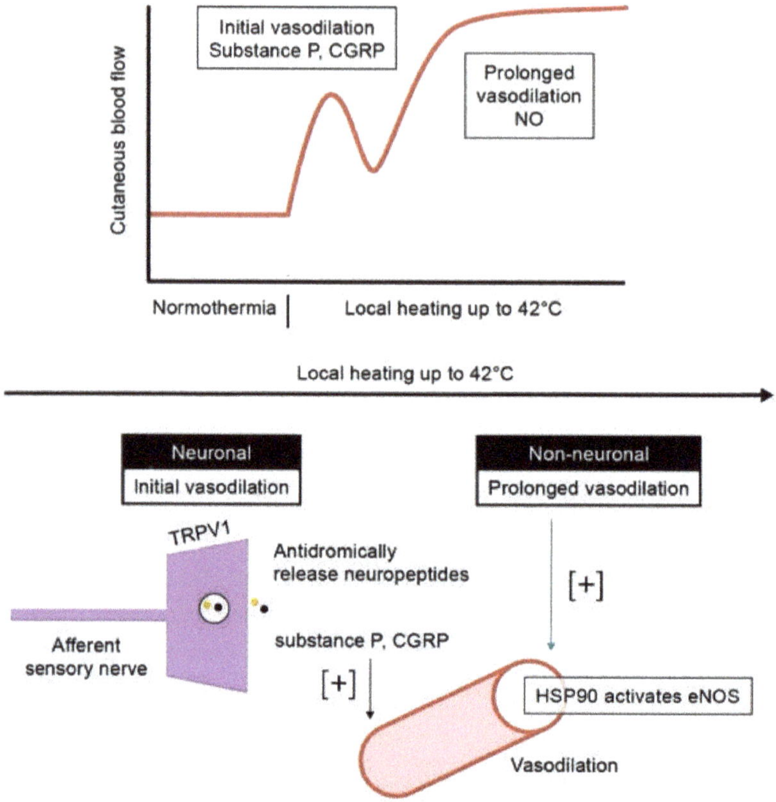


**Figure 85.** Mechanism of vasodilation of local thermal stimulation. Local non-nociceptive thermal stimulation (<42 °C) induces a two-phase vasodilation response in the skin. The first peak represents the activation of TRPV1 in the sensory nerves, which is followed by antidromic release of vasoactive substances, such as substance P and CGRP. As temperature continues to rise, there exists a prolonged vasodilation plateau. This is mediated by NO, which is produced in part by heat shock protein activation inducing the production of nitric oxide synthase in the blood vessel endothelia.

References: (modified from (1) In vivo mechanisms of cutaneous vasodilation and vasoconstriction in humans during thermoregulatory challenges. *J Appl Physiol.* 2006;100(5):1709–1718. (2) Exercise training and cutaneous vasodilator function. *Jpn J Phys Fit Sports Med.* 2017;66:185–193.)

is localized, sensory nerves are activated to begin the antidromic release of vasoactive peptides which cause vasodilation. Persistent vasodilation, which is related to NO, occurs when the skin is heated continuously up to 42 °C.

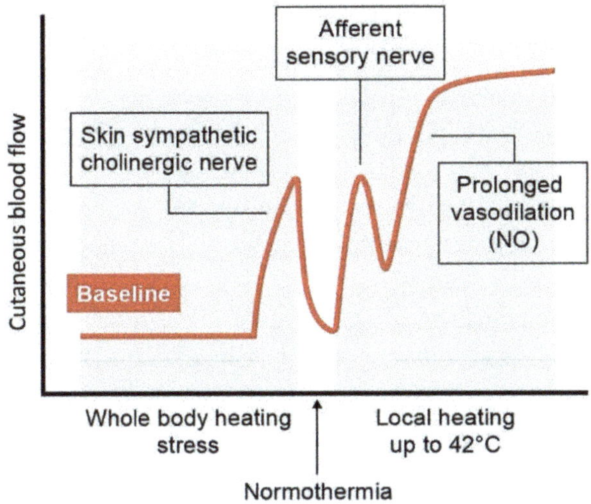


**Figure 86.** Whole body heating and stress (physical or psychological stress) activate the sympathetic cholinergic nerve system in the skin, which in turn causes vasodilation in the cutaneous arterioles. Local non-nociceptive thermal stimulation induces a two-phase vasodilatory response in the skin. The first peak represents the activation of TRPV1 in the sensory nerves, which is followed by antidromic release of vasoactive substances, such as substance P and CGRP. After transient decrease, blood flow gradually increases to a stable plateau. This prolonged vasodilation is associated with the generation of NO.

## 2.20 Nitric oxide and rosacea

Some studies have previously discussed the role of NO in rosacea. Moura and colleagues reported that immunohistochemical analysis of the skin samples from 28 patients with a clinical or pathological diagnosis of rosacea showed a higher expression of inducible nitric oxide synthase (iNOS) than in normal individuals.[34] NOS includes neural NOS (nNOS), endothelial NOS (eNOS), and inducible NOS (iNOS), which can be inhibited by vitamin B12, and particularly, hydroxocobalamin has a strong inhibiting effect on the three types of NOS.[35] Additionally, Cb(II) of hydroxocobalamin is oxidized by NO to become Cb(III), which forms a covalent bond with NO to create a ligand.[36]

Based on the fact that the levels of iNOS in the facial skin are higher in patients with rosacea than normal individuals, theoretically, NO is somehow involved in the persistent rosacea erythema. Continued non-nociceptive thermal stimulation leads to a prolonged vasodilation, which involves NO.[29–31] Hydroxocobalamin, a form of vitamin B12, exhibits a strong inhibitory effect on NOS, further reducing vasodilation caused by NO. Our study evaluates the effects of hydroxocobalamin on persistent erythema and facial flushing in patients with rosacea. The results of this study were published in the Journal of Clinical and Aesthetic Dermatology by Dr. Huang Yi-Wei, Dr. Huang Hui-Peng, Prof. Hsu Chao-Kai, and Prof. Lee Yu-Yun.[37]

Our study involved the observation of 13 patients with rosacea who experienced persistent erythema or facial flushing, and hydroxocobalamin was weekly administered to the participants at a dose of 1–2 mg via intramuscular injection, and such treatment lasted for 1–4 weeks. We used two assessment methods: first, the CEA grade of the patients, and second, the surface temperature of the skin taken via infrared thermometer. We compared the difference in the skin of the cheeks before and after treatment.

Thirty minutes after the first hydroxocobalamin injection was administered, the mean CEA grade decreased from 2.2 ± 0.6 to 1.2 ± 0.4 ($p < 0.001$) (Figure 87), and the cheek surface temperature decreased from 36.7 ± 0.70 °C to 36.2 ± 0.61 °C ($p < 0.001$) (Figure 88). The results demonstrate that injection of hydroxocobalamin results in the immediate

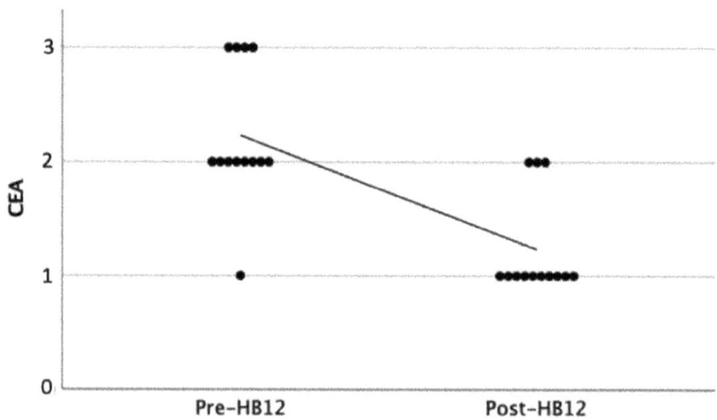


**Figure 87.** The effect of hydroxocobalamin on persistent erythema and facial flushing in patients with rosacea shows a reduction in the mean grade of Clinician's Erythema Assessment (CEA) from 2.2 ± 0.6 to 1.2 ± 0.4 (n = 13, $p < 0.001$). HB12, Hydroxocobalamin; *$p < 0.001$. (Source: *J Clin Aesthet Dermatol.* 2022;15(6):42–45).

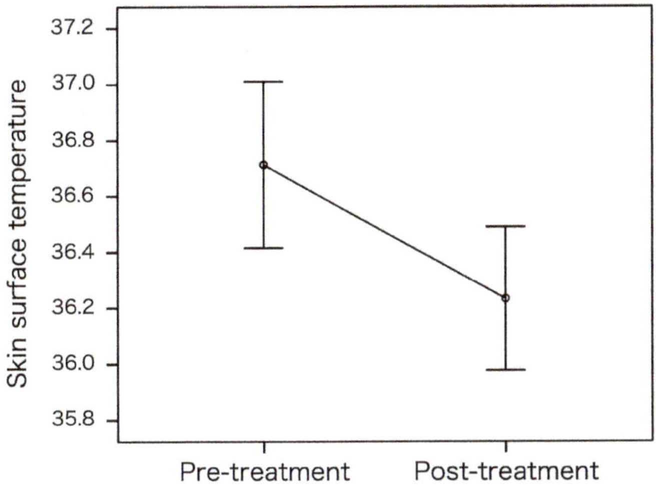


**Figure 88.** Reduction of skin surface temperature of the cheek in patients with rosacea treated with hydroxocobalamin (n = 24 treatments). $*p < 0.001$.

Reference: *J Clin Aesthet Dermatol.* 2022;15(6):42–45.

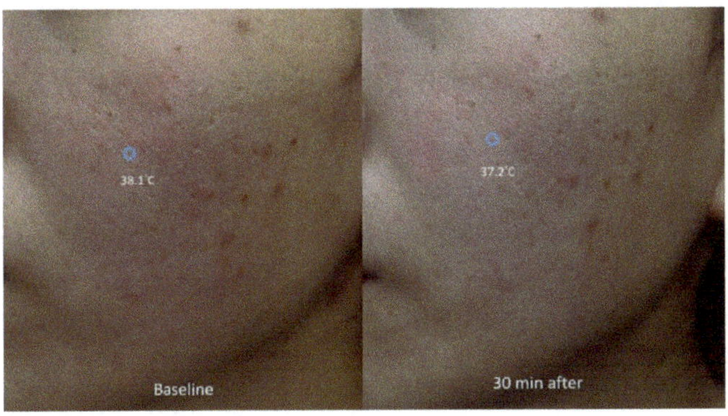


**Figure 89.** Intramuscular injection of 1-mg hydroxocobalamin. Comparing pretreatment with 30 minutes post-treatment, facial erythema is visibly reduced and the skin temperature dropped by 0.8 °C.

Reference: J Clin Aesthet Dermatol. 2022;15(6):42–45.

relief of erythema in patients with rosacea (Figure 89). Patients also perceived that their persistent facial flushing was either no longer present or had been significantly reduced and shortened in duration. However, one patient with erythema showed a slight flare.[37]

## 2.21 Treating rosacea erythema and flushing with botulinum toxin A

In 2004, Yuraitis and Jacob were the first to report a case in which botulinum toxin A (hereinafter referred to as BoNT-A) was injected to treat the facial flushing symptoms associated with rosacea. Ten units of BoNT-A (manufactured by Allergan plc), diluted to 2 U/0.1 mL, were injected into the dermal–subdermal interface of one cheek at 1-cm intervals.[38] In 2005, a case was reported in which a patient developed a severe droop of the right cheek and upper lip after receiving BoNT-A injections into the dermal–subdermal interface. In the case, the right cheek was selectively injected and the BoNT-A was diluted to a concentration of 4 U/0.1 mL. Four injections were administered at 1-cm intervals, with 2 U of BoNT-A given at each site.[39] It was not until 2015 that the use of BoNT-A to treat rosacea was reported in the literature. In a South Korean study, two patients with rosacea were injected with BoNT-A at 90 degrees intradermally. The concentration, dosage, and interval were all the same as those in the 2004 report. However, a second BoNT-A injection was administered every other week. By a week after the second treatment, the researchers observed significant improvements in erythema and facial flushing, and the patients were satisfied with their physical appearance. No significant side effects were reported, and only slight pain and localized bruising were experienced during the treatment.[40]

Currently, there are various BoNT-A products on the market, and therapeutic dosages differ depending on the amount of core protein within the unit. Dysport (Abobotulinumtoxin A) 17 U, Botox (Onabotulinumtoxin A) 10 U, and Xeomin (Incobotulinumtoxin A) 22.5 U require 0.09 ng of core protein.[41] Another Merzu-related study reported active core protein levels of 0.44 ng for Dysport 500U, Botox 100U, and Xeomin 100U.[42] However, our years of experience working with Dysport and Botox make it difficult to agree with the latter report.

The efficacy of Korean brands such as Prabotulinumtoxin A (Nabota) does not differ substantially from that of Botox.[43] BoNT-A can improve the facial flushing mechanism because heat or stress will stimulate the sympathetic cholinergic nerve fibers, resulting in the release of vesicles from the nerve endings. These vesicles from sympathetic cholinergic nerve contain acetylcholine and other cotransmitters.

However, acetylcholine is not the primary substance causing the dilation of arterioles in the skin, but rather other cotransmitters.[29] Because the sympathetic nerve reaction stimulated by heat or stress is stronger in patients with rosacea than normal individuals, this results in the appearance of the erythema and flushing associated with rosacea.[29,30,33] Stress stimulation includes both psychological and physiological stress. The former is when the patient is subjected to an arithmetic test in which the patient is asked to consecutively subtract 7 or 11 for 1–2 minutes, whereas the latter is when the patient is subjected to an isometric hand grip test for 1–2 minutes.[33] BoNT-A is able to inhibit the release of vesicles from the sympathetic cholinergic nerve and sensory nerve,[44,45] thus improving symptoms. We can use the arithmetic test and the isometric hand grip test to clinically screen patients suitable for the treatment of rosacea using BoNT-A. Patients with visible stress-associated facial flushing before treatment can undergo intradermal BoNT-A injection treatment. The maximal effect appeared 2–3 weeks after treatment in my patients taking serial arithmetic test. The patients took the arithmetic and isometric hand grip tests again to assess the sympathetic cholinergic flushing of the skin, which either no longer occurs or is significantly reduced. For patients in whom sympathetic flushing has not been completely eliminated, a second session of intradermal BoNT-A injection treatment may be considered. However, neurogenic rosacea is more unpredictable as to whether injections will be effective or result in short-term side effects; thus, special attention should be paid to the use of BoNT-A injections. The management of neurogenic rosacea is described in Section 3.4.2.

In addition to the aforementioned study, another study with a larger sample size analyzed the results of using Dysport to treat erythema and facial flushing in 15 patients. After 3 months of observation, 6/15 patients showed improved symptoms after 1 month of treatment, and 11/15 patients showed improved symptoms after 3 months.[46]

In 2019, Dr. Kim's team published a randomized, double-blind, and placebo-controlled split-face study to evaluate the physiological changes and safety of skin after the intradermal injection of BoNT-A in patients with facial rosacea erythema. Twenty-four participants showed a significant decrease in the CEA grade of the side of the face treated with *Clostridium botulinum*, as well as a significant increase on the global aesthetic improvement scale, a decrease on the erythema index in the fourth and eighth weeks, improvements in skin elasticity in the second and fourth weeks, and a significant improvement in skin hydration in the second, fourth, and eighth weeks. However, transepidermal water loss and sebum secretion had no significant difference.[47] In addition, there are reported cases of BoNT-A being used together with pulsed light or Tixel (Thermal Mechanical Action) to treat erythema and facial flushing in patients with rosacea.[48,49] Research has shown that BoNT-A combined with Tixel can have effects which last up to 6 months.[48]

BoNT-A is used in the treatment of rosacea in the same way as in the treatment of other conditions, and may cause side effects. Injections must avoid the modiolus, as this is the area where the muscle fibers used to control expression enter the dermis. In a case recorded in Taiwan, papules broke out after the injection of BoNT. It is important to note the angle of injection. The authors recommend that injections are performed at an approximate angle of 30°–45°, but the small injection angle may cause the drug to be squeezed out of the injection site.

In summary, BoNT can be used to treat the symptoms of erythema and facial flushing in patients with rosacea. The total dosage for both cheeks should be diluted from 20 U to 1 cc (Botox), with 5 U added to the midpoint and injected intradermally. The effects will become visible approximately 1 day to 1 month after the injection and will last for 3–6 months. In terms of reactions to the injection, most patients experience an improvement in their erythema or facial flushing. Patients with neurogenic rosacea may exhibit anxiety, nervousness, and distrust. Initial treatment with gabapentinoids and TCA may lead to some improvement in stinging and burning sensations, which help build the patient's trust. Follow-up treatment with Botulinum toxin A can further ease the treatment course.

## 2.22 Dr. Huang's dual antiheat treatment for erythema and flushing of rosacea

Dr Huang's dual antiheat treatment for rosacea erythema and flushing is a combination of BoNT-A and hydroxocobalamin, which is used to treat both erythema and facial flushing. BoNT is used to inhibit the abnormal facial skin sympathetic cholinergic and afferent sensory activity induced by heat and stress, and hydroxocobalamin acts as an NO scavenger.

### 2.22.1 *Nitric oxide scavenger: hydroxocobalamin*

Nitric oxide (NO) may facilitate the release of CGRP from afferent nerve fibers or be a secondary vasorelaxant messenger of the peptide.[1] NO is a mediator of skin sympathetic cholinergic nerve.[2]

Furthermore, NO also is the primary mediator of prolonged vasodilation.[3] Moreover, NO is a regulator of mast cell activation and mast cell-mediated inflammation.[4]

Vitamin B12 hydroxocobalamin acts as the NO scavenger to form ligands, capturing excess NO in the background of rosacea skin, which alleviates persistent erythema and even binds to the NO produced by localized prolonged thermal stimulation to inhibit the prolonged vasodilation and flushing caused by NO. This is particularly significant for patients who engage in intense exercise or who work in kitchens and represents a major improvement in quality of life. Visible effects can be seen 30 minutes after intramuscular injection of hydroxocobalamin, with optimal effects persisting for 2–6 days (Figure 90). Some patients with rosacea had stabilized and almost invisible erythema a few months after being administered with hydroxocobalamin (Figure 91). For patients with rosacea and burning sensation possibly caused by mast cell overactivity, Vitamin B12 use may exacerbate erythema and flushing.

### 2.22.2 *BoNT-A inhibits skin sympathetic cholinergic nerves*

BoNT-A inhibits the release of cotransmitters from the vesicles of the cholinergic branch of the sympathetic nerves, and inhibits sympathetic flushing.[29,30] In other words, the sympathetic response caused by systemic thermal stimulation or by physiological or psychological stress is blocked. Patients with rosacea have stronger skin sympathetic response than control participants.[33] The inhibition of sympathetic flushing by BoNT is understandable and verifiable by the fact that sympathetic flushing is visibly stopped or reduced in patients with rosacea subjected to arithmetic and isometric hand grip tests before and after BoNT treatment. BoNT-A has been verified to reduce the expression of TRPV1 in sensory nerve endings and has been shown to reduce erythema in patients with rosacea (Figure 92),[50,51] the exact reasons for which are unknown. It is possible that the sympathetic

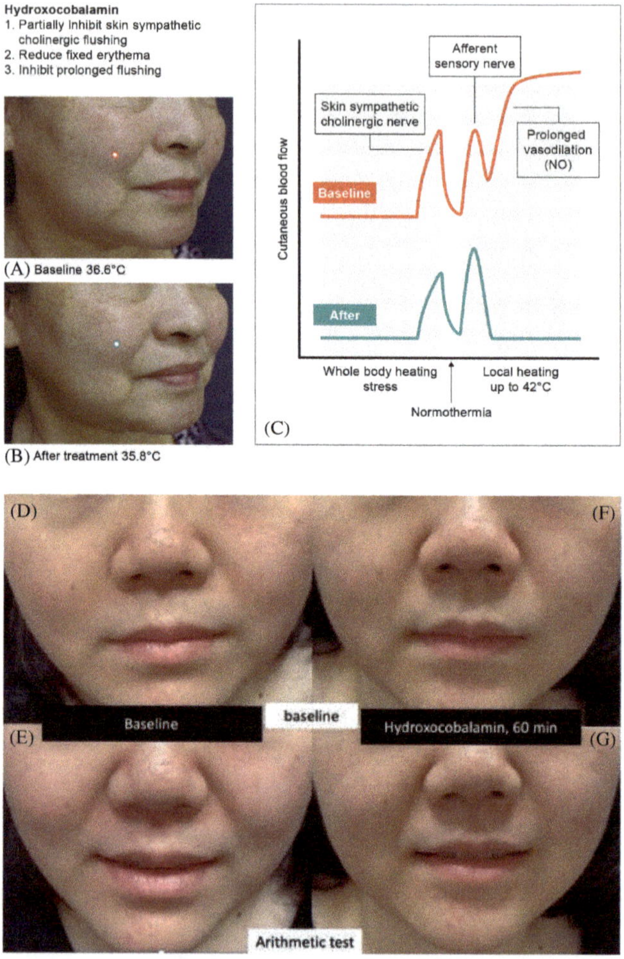


**Figure 90.** Treatment for rosacea erythema and facial flushing with hydroxocobalamin. Erythema was alleviated 30 minutes after intramuscular injection of 1-mg hydroxocobalamin (A, B). Hydroxocobalamin increased heat tolerance to avoid the prolonged facial flushing caused by prolonged heating. The red simulated curve represents the pretreatment conditions, whereas the green curve represents post-treatment conditions (C). Hydroxocobalamin treatment also reduced skin flushing caused by arithmetic test that activating skin sympathetic cholinergic vasodilation (D–G). Fixed erythema was alleviated after the application of hydroxocobalamin. Facial flushing is less severe during the arithmetic test after treatment than before treatment, indicating that NO is a factor in skin sympathetic cholinergic flushing.

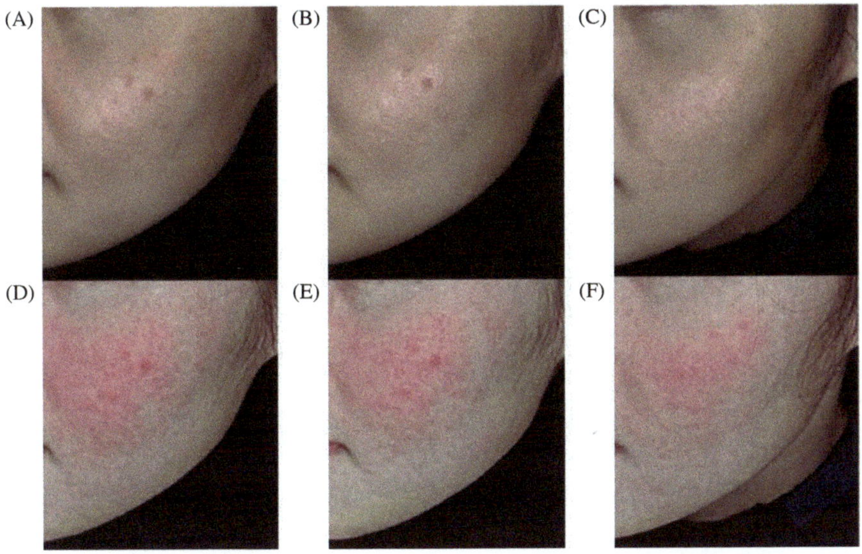


**Figure 91.** Topical hydroxocobalamin and changes in erythema. Skin pretreatment conditions (A, D) versus 35 minutes post-treatment (B, E). An immediate alleviation in erythema can be seen. After 3.5 months of continuous use (C, F), erythema is stabilized and almost undetectable. OBSERV skin analysis technology in natural light (A–C), Erythema Index (D–F).

cholinergic nerves of patients with rosacea are often in a state of excitation. The effect of BoNT in the arteries is to inhibit vasoconstriction,[52,53] which is insufficient to explain the alleviation of persistent erythema.

### 2.22.3 *Hydroxocobalamin combined with BoNT-A*

The treatment results of vitamin B12 hydroxocobalamin combined with BoNT-A demonstrate that intramuscular injection of 1-mg hydroxocobalamin reduces facial skin temperature by 0.5 °C in 30 minutes post-treatment (Figure 88), whereas intramuscular 1-mg hydroxocobalamin combined with intradermal BoNT-A (Botox) reduces facial skin temperature by 1 °C–1.4 °C (Table 10) by the following day. This indicates a clear improvement in results (Figure 93). In response to thermal and stress stimulation, sensory nerve flushing remains the same or is diminished, but skin sympathetic flushing and persistent flushing are almost completely eliminated, and improvements in persistent erythema are more pronounced than in patients

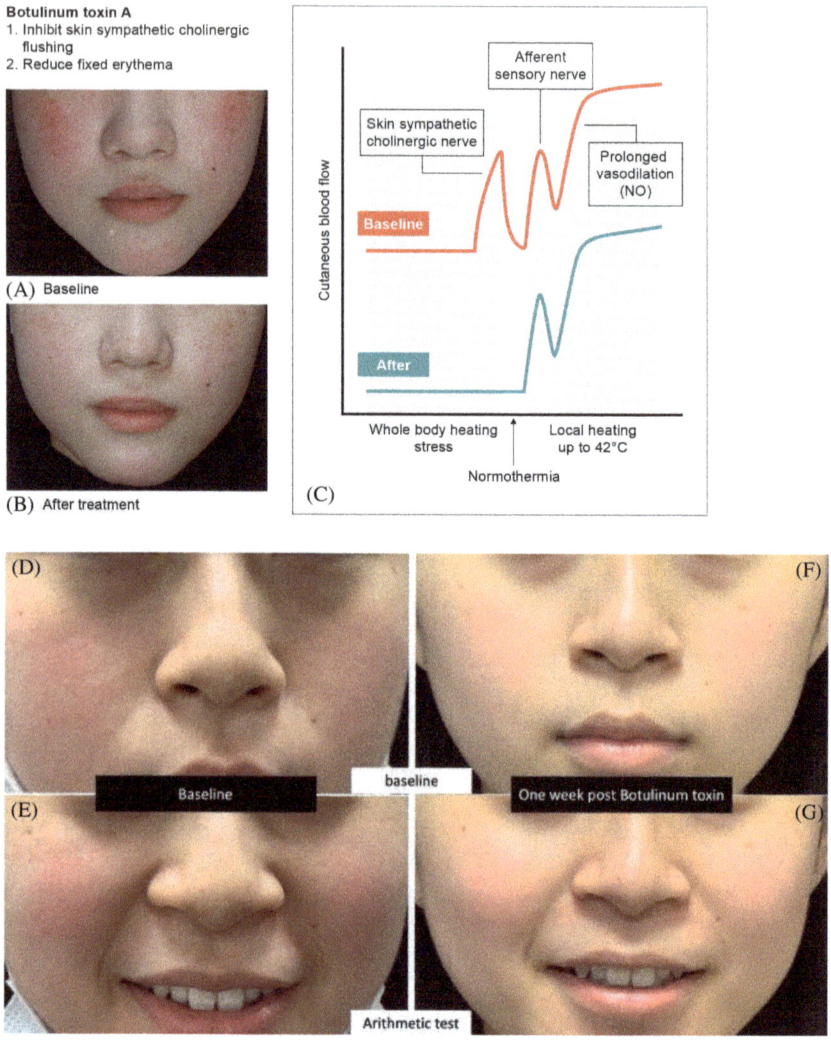


**Figure 92.** Treatment for rosacea erythema and facial flushing with botulinum toxin A (BoNT-A). Erythema was reduced one week after intradermal injection of BoNT-A (A, B). BoNT-A inhibits sympathetic cholinergic flushing of the skin. The red simulated curve represents pretreatment conditions; the green curve represents post-treatment conditions(C). Record of erythema during arithmetic test showed reduction in fixed erythema and facial flushing after BoNT-A treatment (D–G).

**Table 10.** Clinical data of 16 rosacea patients treated with hydroxocobalamin intramuscular and botulinum toxin intradermal injection

| Case | Age | Sex | Presentation | Pre-treatment | Post-treatment | HB12 dose/sessions | Botolnum toxin dose/sessions | CEA | CEA* | Follow up |
|---|---|---|---|---|---|---|---|---|---|---|
| 1 | 50 | F | Erythema, flushing | Methylcobalamin Levocetirizine Metronidazole gel | (Methylcobalamin Levocetirizine) x 1 week | 1 mg/1 | Botox 20, 22U/ 5.5months apart | 3 | 0–1 | Stable at 9th month |
| 2 | 62 | F | Erythema, flushing, burning, itching | Pulsed dye laser, levocetirizine 3 weeks ago | None | 1 mg /3 | Botox 20U, 20U, 20U/ one month then 3 months apart | 2 | 0–1 | |
| 3 | 39 | M | Erythema, flushing Seborrheic dermatitis | None in the past 2 months | None | 2mg/2 Then topical HB12 for one month | Botox 20U, 20U, 20U/2 weeks then 7 months apart | 3 | 1–2 | |
| 4 | 55 | F | Erythema, flushing | Methylcobalamin 500μg tid Isotretinoin 20mg qd | None | 1–2mg/4 | Botox 20U, 20U/10 days apart | 3 | 1–2 | Stable at 9th month |
| 5 | 45 | F | Erythema, flushing | None | None | 1mg/2 | Botox 20U once | 3 | 1 | |
| 6 | 45 | F | Erythema, flushing | None | None | 1mg/3 | Botox 25U once | 3 | 2 | |

(*Continued*)

**Table 10.** *(Continued)*

| Case | Age | Sex | Presentation | Pre-treatment | Post-treatment | HB12 dose/sessions | Botolnum toxin dose/ sessions | CEA | CEA* | Follow up |
|---|---|---|---|---|---|---|---|---|---|---|
| 7 | 35 | F | Erythema, flushing, (Demodex overgrowth) | (Topical ivermectin, Carvedilol, fexodine, methylcobal) x 1 week | Topical ivermectin, Carvedilol, fexodine | 1–2mg/3 | Botox 20U once | 2 | 2 | 3 weeks |
| 8 | 40 | F | Erythema, flushing | Carvedilol, methylcobalamin | None | 1–2mg/5 | Botox 20U, 20U, 20U, 20U/3, 1, 3 months apart | 3 | 1 | 8 months |
| 9 | 39 | F | Erythema, flushing | Isotretinoin 20mg qod, levocetirizine | Pregabalin, carvedilol, isotretinoin | 1–2mg/3 | Botox 25U once | 2 | 1 | |
| 10 | 63 | M | Erythema, flushing | (Carvedilol, Methylcobalamin) x 2 months | Carvedilol | 1–2mg/4 | Botox 25U, 25U/ 2 weeks apart | 3 | 1–2 | 3 weeks |
| 11 | 33 | F | Erythema, flushing (Demodex overgrowth) | None | Topical ivermectin | 2mg/ 3 Methylcobalamin x 60 days | Botox 20U, 20U, 20U/ 1 week, 3 weeks apart | 2 | 1 | Stable at 9th month |
| 12 | 41 | F | Erythema, flushing | Doxycycline, metronidazole gel | Isotretinoin, carvedilol | | Botox 20U, 25U/ 1 week apart | 1–2 | 1 | |

| | | | | | | | | | |
|---|---|---|---|---|---|---|---|---|---|
| 13 | 44 | F | Erythema, flushing | None | | HB12 500ug bid x 4 weeks | Botox 20U, 20U/1 week apart | 2 | 1 | 5 months |
| 14 | 59 | F | Erythema, flushing, burning | oral ivermectin, flunarizine, carvedilol, oral metronidazole, plaquenil, stilnox for 2 years. | Pregabalin adds to the prior medications. Carvedilol was added at 2nd month. | Worsen post HB12 1mg im | Botox 25U once | 3–4 | 2→3→1 | |
| 15 | 49 | F | Erythema, flushing | Methylcobalamin for 9 months | None | Oral or topical HB12 | Botox 25U, 25U, 25U/ 2 weeks then 4months apart | 3 | 1 | |
| 16 | 46 | F | Erythema, flushing (Demodex overgrowth) | Topical ivermectin | Topical ivermectin | topical HB12 | Letybo 25U, Botox 25U/ 3 weeks apart | 2 | 1 | |

HB12, hydroxocobalamin.

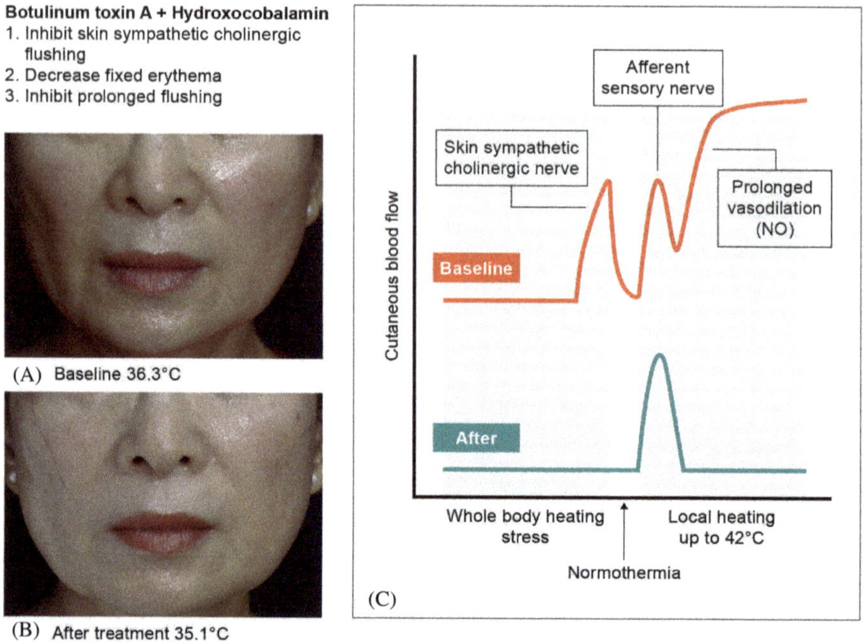


**Figure 93.** Treatment for rosacea with hydroxocobalamin combined with BoNT-A. There was a pronounced improvement of facial flushing and erythema (A, B). Skin sympathetic cholinergic flushing and prolonged flushing are decreased. The red simulated curve represents pretreatment conditions, and the green curve represents post-treatment conditions (C).

administered with the individual treatment. With repeated sessions of intradermal BoNT-A treatment the afferent sensory flushing induced by hair dryer blowing can be eliminated.

In clinical case observations, approximately 1/13 patients with rosacea experience flaring up of their erythema after hydroxocobalamin treatment, whereas 50% of patients with neurogenic rosacea and experiencing burning or prickling sensation will have their symptoms worsened by hydroxocobalamin. These individuals may initially experience good results, but after several days to approximately 2 weeks, negative reactions will develop. BoNT treatment for neurogenic rosacea may result in temporary deterioration of symptoms, followed by an improvement. The pretreatment arithmetic and isometric grip strength tests are useful in screening patients with rosacea for BoNT treatment. The individual

**Table 11.** Dr Huang's dual antiheat treatment for rosacea erythema and flushing

| | Intramuscular hydroxocobalamin | Intradermal botulinum toxin A |
|---|---|---|
| Dose | 1–2 mg | 20–25U (Botox) |
| Onset | 30 minutes | 1 day to 1 month |
| Peak | 30 minutes to 1 hour | Usually 2–3 weeks |
| Duration Results | 2–6 days | 3–6 months |

recommended doses, onset of efficacy times, peak times, and duration of hydroxocobalamin and BoNT-A are shown in Table 11.

Theoretically, topical administration of hydroxocobalamin is superior to systemic administration, and NO is necessary for many physiological functions, such as the erectile function of the male sex organ. The frequency of BoNT injections can range from 1 week to 1 month depending on the patient's clinical response or reaction to the arithmetic test, and optimal results can typically be maintained for 3–6 months.

Sensory nerve flushing is the current challenge in the treatment of rosacea erythema and flushing. In a sensory neuron cell culture study, BoNT-A inhibited the KCL-induced secretion of substance P and CGRP.[54] However, in 1995, Kellogg's team demonstrated that localized thermal stimulation induces sensory nerve vasodilation unaffected by BoNT.[29] The mechanism of sensory nerve flushing is the activation of small C fibers by localized non-nociceptive thermal stimulation or capsaicin via TRPV1 and by cold stimulation via TRPA1. This is followed by the antidromic release of vasoactive peptides substance P and CGRP, which in turn results in vasodilation and flushing.[29,55] Patients with rosacea who undergo BoNT-A treatment continue to experience flushing when wearing a face mask, indicating that localized thermal stimulation still activates the vasodilation of sensory nerves.

## 2.23 Breaking the curse for patients with rosacea who love exercise

According to Yamazaki, an increase in core body temperature during persistent exercise inhibits the cutaneous adrenergic sympathetic vasoconstriction system and activates the skin sympathetic cholinergic vasodilation system. In addition, local skin temperature will increase, which activates the vasodilatory response of sensory nerves and NO.[53] Dr. Huang's proposed heat-resistant treatment for rosacea means that the rapid reduction of erythema and flushing in patients with rosacea is now increasingly attainable. It can increase the level of heat resistance in the skin of those with rosacea and cause erythema and flushing to fade rapidly. This is an innovative approach and a boon for those with rosacea who enjoy engaging in exercise. For these individuals, exercise is no longer restricted to indoors or underwater and can involve outdoor exercise, ball games, hot yoga, running outdoors, and any other exercise activities the individual enjoys.

### 2.23.1 *An exercise-loving woman with rosacea*

A 56-year-old woman who loves to exercise, particularly jogging and brisk walks, had her rosacea flared up by the increased intensity and frequency of her exercise. She reported that the skin on her face would develop flushing and a burning sensation after exercise and would take a long time to subside, to the extent that she would have to use air conditioning and an electric fan to blow cold air on her skin as well as apply an ice pack for around 40 minutes before her skin returned to its prior condition (Figure 94). We started treatment with topical tranexamic acid and hydroxocobalamin treatment.

⑩ An excerpt of pretreatment interview:

Dr. Huang: "Could you please explain what circumstances usually cause your facial flushing?"

Patient: "If I have been for a long walk and I return to a hot and stifling environment where air conditioning has been turned off, it will lead to my facial flushing. I have been exercising more often recently. I started by running 5 km in a day, but now after running slowly each day for over a week, my T-zone has become much more severe than usual. I suspect that the exercise caused it to become unstable."

Dr. Huang: "What do you do to bring the temperature down in case of facial flushing?"

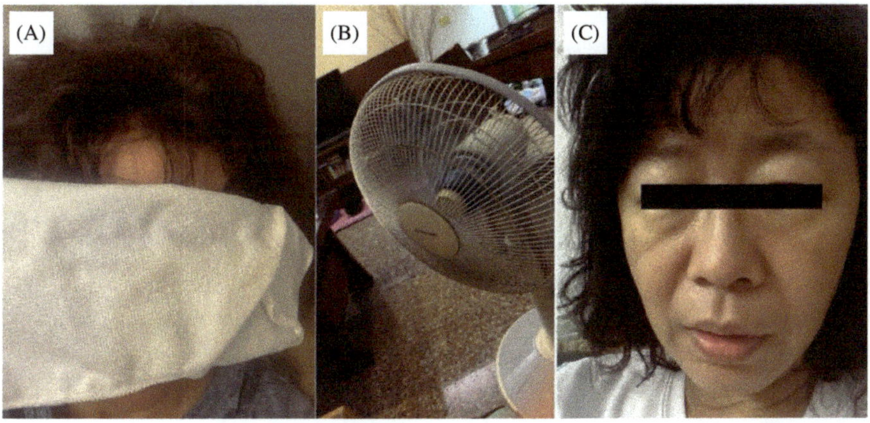


**Figure 94.** (A), (B), (C) A female patient with rosacea experienced facial burning and flushing after long exercise routine, and these symptoms subsided after using air-conditioning, electric fan, and cold packing for 10 minutes.

Patient: "I did not do anything for my facial flushing. But later on, I began to feel a tingling sensation in my skin, i.e., the tingling sensation became more pronounced under normal conditions without doing any exercise, and my skin felt rough to the touch. Subsequently, I started to cool my skin after exercise. I would wrap a bag of ice in a towel as an ice pack to make cold compress and then use an electric fan to blow cold air, and I would sometimes spray water in the cold air too. This was enough to bring the temperature down."

Dr. Huang: "When you use the ice pack and blow cold air, how long would it take to bring the temperature down?"

Patient: "It depends on the exercise intensity. Yesterday, I was walking at a brisk pace, so about 1 km every 10 minutes, and I think it took around 10 minutes to bring down the temperature subsequently, but that was with brisk walking and no running."

Dr. Huang: "And that was with both cold air and an ice pack?"

Patient: "Yes!"

Dr. Huang: "If you didn't blow the cold air or use the ice pack, how long do you think it would take to bring down the temperature?"

Patient: "I think it would take around 40–50 minutes, because that was without air conditioning."

Dr. Huang: "And when you're in the kitchen, is this..."

Patient: "Yes, it is the same! I had no idea why I had facial flushing in the past, particularly when I fry fish and when the frying pan is hot, my face feels very uncomfortable, with flushing and burning."

⑩ The effects of topical tranexamic acid and hydroxocobalamin treatment

We conducted a clinical observation of the effects of topical tranexamic acid and hydroxocobalamin treatment.

Purpose: To assess the efficacy of the treatment in improving facial temperature, erythema, and flushing.

Method: We measured the cheek temperature and took photographs (Canon EOS 750D and OBSERV 520x). These were used to assess the effects of administering topical tranexamic and hydroxocobalamin treatment. Forty minutes after administration, we again measured cheek temperature and photographed it. Next, we used a blow dryer to blow warm air onto the face and hair for 2 minutes and measured the cheek temperature and photographed it again. Subsequently, the air conditioning was switched off and the patient was asked to run in an enclosed room for 10 minutes. We measured cheek temperature once again, and took another photograph.

Results: The post-treatment OBSERV 520x erythema image assessment revealed a decrease in erythema after 40 minutes. Centrofacial erythema was further reduced 60 minutes after the face was heated with warm air for 2 minutes, with only a small area of flushing on the chin. The erythema at 84 minutes, after running on the spot, was unchanged from the erythema at 60 minutes. Comparison of the skin temperature at each measurement and the image of the erythema is shown in Figure 95.

Three weeks after treatment, we conducted another interview. Dr. Huang: "Could you tell me about any changes you have noticed since your treatment?" Patient: "When I first rub the reparative serum on my skin, it feels a little cold and tight, but then I can go about my day as normal. Moreover, when I exercise, my face is less likely to react seriously by flushing and swelling. After I run, my face is less tingly, less burning, and less flushing than it used to be." (Figure 96).

| Skin surface temperature (°C) | Baseline | After 40min | After 60 min (post hair dryer blowing for 2 minutes) | After 84 min (Post running in place for 10 minutes) |
|---|---|---|---|---|
| Left cheek | 36.2 | 35.7 | 36.3 | 36.6 |
| Right cheek | 36.1 | 35.6 | 35.9 | 36.3 |
| Forehead | 36.4 | 36.1 | 35.9 | 36.3 |
| Chin | 36.4 | 36.1 | 36.1 | 36.1 |
| Erythema index (Observ R1 value) | 0.1983 | 0.1762 | 0.1988 | 0.1553 |

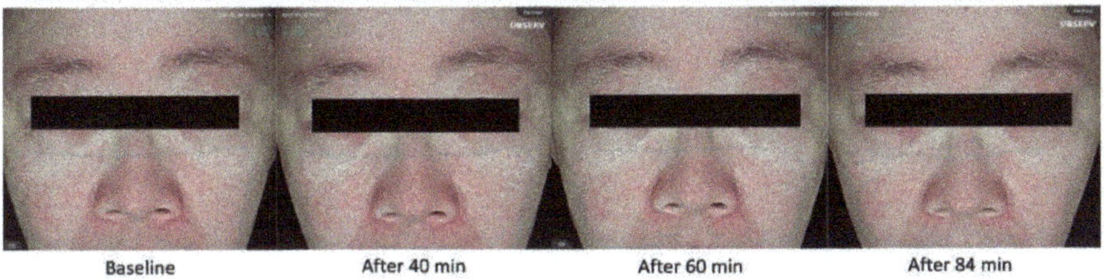


**Figure 95.** The effects of topical tranexamic acid and hydroxocobalamin treatment for rosacea. A reduction in skin surface temperature, erythema, and flushing was observed at different time points after application of the topical cream.

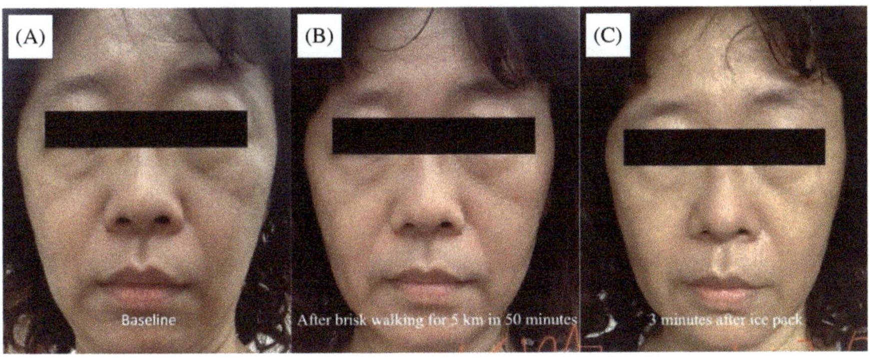


**Figure 96.** A, B, C. The topical tranexamic acid and hydroxocobalamin treatment were conducted for 3 weeks. The treatment was administered at around 9 am, and the patient exercised at around 5 pm; after running, the patient reported less tingling, heat, and flushing in the skin, and flushing subsided much faster than prior to treatment.

## 2.24 Immediate response of treatment for erythema, covering neurovascular response mechanisms

As the sub-pathways of rosacea have been illustrated, some topical products with active ingredients inhibiting targets of rosacea are potentially in the future (Figure 97).

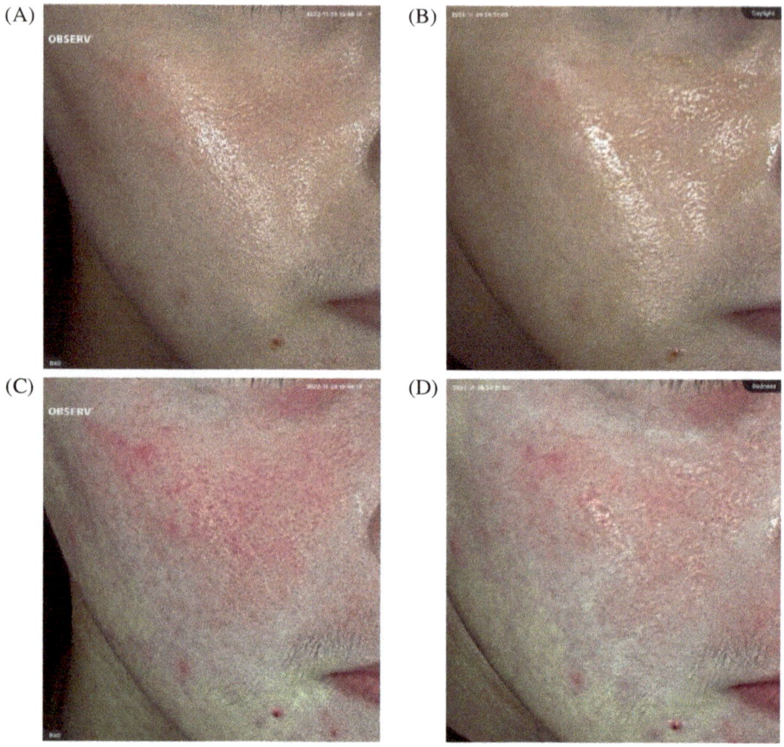


**Figure 97.** Effects of treatment on rosacea erythema and flushing, covering neurovascular response mechanisms. Using the OBSERV skin scanner with natural light: (A) Prior to treatment and (B) 45 minutes post-treatment. Facial erythema index: (C) Prior to treatment and (D) 45 minutes post-treatment.

## References

1. Huang HP, Hsu CK, Lee JY. A new superficial needle-scraping method for assessing *Demodex* density in papulopustular rosacea. *J Cosmet Dermatol.* 2020;19(4):896–900.
2. Huang HP, Hsu CK, Lee JY. Thumbnail-squeezing method: an effective method for assessing *Demodex* density in rosacea. *J Eur Acad Dermatol Venereol.* 2020;34(7):e343–e345.
3. Forton FM, De Maertelaer V. Two consecutive standardized skin surface biopsies: an improved sampling method to evaluate *Demodex* density as a

diagnostic tool for rosacea and demodicosis. *Acta Derm Venereol.* 2017;97(2):242–248.

4. Turgut Erdemir A, Gurel MS, Koku Aksu AE, Falay T, Inan Yuksel E, Sarikaya E. *Demodex* mites in acne rosacea: reflectance confocal microscopic study. *Australas J Dermatol.* 2017;58(2):e26–e30.
5. Chen W, Plewig G. Human demodicosis: revisit and a proposed classification. *Br J Dermatol.* 2014;170(6):1219–1225.
6. Taieb A, Ortonne JP, Ruzicka T, et al. Superiority of ivermectin 1% cream over metronidazole 0.75% cream in treating inflammatory lesions of rosacea: a randomized, investigator-blinded trial. *Br J Dermatol.* 2015;172(4):1103–1110.
7. Huang H P, Hsu CK, Lee J Y. Rosacea with persistent facial erythema and high *Demodex* density effectively treated with topical ivermectin alone or combined with oral carvedilol. *Dermatol Ther.* 2021;34(2):e14899.
8. Taieb A, Khemis A, Ruzicka T, et al. Maintenance of remission following successful treatment of papulopustular rosacea with ivermectin 1% cream vs. metronidazole 0.75% cream: 36-week extension of the ATTRACT randomized study. *J Eur Acad Dermatol Venereol.* 2016;30(5):829–836.
9. Trave I, Merlo G, Cozzani E, Parodi A. Real-life experience on effectiveness and tolerability of topical ivermectin in papulopustular rosacea and antiparasitic effect on *Demodex* mites. *Dermatol Ther.* 2019;32(6):e13093.
10. Schaller M, Gonser L, Belge K, et al. Dual anti-inflammatory and antiparasitic action of topical ivermectin 1% in papulopustular rosacea. *J Eur Acad Dermatol Venereol.* 2017;31(11):1907–1911.
11. Zhang J, Jiang P, Sheng L, et al. A novel mechanism of carvedilol efficacy for rosacea treatment: toll-like receptor 2 inhibition in macrophages. *Front Immunol.* 2021;12:609615.
12. Eckert MM, Gundin NL. Treatment of rosacea with topical ivermectin cream: a series of 34 cases. *Dermatol Online J.* 2016;22(8).
13. Koller B, Müller-Wiefel AS, Rupec R, Korting HC, Ruzicka T. Chitin modulates innate immune responses of keratinocytes. *PLoS One.* 2011;6(2): e16594.
14. McMahon F, Banville N, Bergin DA, et al. Activation of neutrophils via IP3 pathway following exposure to *Demodex*-associated bacterial proteins. *Inflammation.* 2016;39(1):425–433.
15. Lacey N, Delaney S, Kavanagh K, Powell FC. Mite-related bacterial antigens stimulate inflammatory cells in rosacea. *Br J Dermatol.* 2007;157(3):474–481.

16. Huang HP, Hsu CK, Lee JY. Topical ivermectin-induced transient flare of rosacea as a host reaction to killed *Demodex* mites preventable by short-term use of topical corticosteroid. *Dermatol Ther.* 2022;35(7):e15517.
17. Gao YY, Di Pascuale MA, Li W, et al. High prevalence of *Demodex* in eyelashes with cylindrical dandruff. *Invest Ophthalmol Vis Sci.* 2005;46(9):3089–3094.
18. Murphy O, O'Dwyer V, Lloyd-McKernan A. Ocular *Demodex folliculorum*: prevalence and associated symptoms in an Irish population. *Int Ophthalmol.* 2019;39(2):405–417.
19. Forton FMN, De Maertelaer V. Rosacea and demodicosis: little-known diagnostic signs and symptoms. *Acta Derm Venereol.* 2019;99(1):47–52.
20. Segal R, Mimouni D, Feuerman H, Pagovitz O, David M. Dermoscopy as a diagnostic tool in demodicidosis. *Int J Dermatol.* 2010;49(9):1018–1023.
21. Friedman P, Sabban EC, Cabo H. Usefulness of dermoscopy in the diagnosis and monitoring treatment of demodicidosis. *Dermatol Pract Concept.* 2017;7(1):35–38.
22. Errichetti E, Figini M, Galvan A. *Demodex* tails on dermoscopy beyond demodicosis: another pitfall to avoid. *Int J Dermatol.* 2021;60(10):e405–e407.
23. Tan ST, Bialostocki A, Armstrong JR. Pulsed dye laser therapy for rosacea. *Br J Plast Surg.* 2004;57(4):303–310.
24. Bernstein EF, Schomacker K, Paranjape A, Jones CJ. Pulsed dye laser treatment of rosacea using a novel 15 mm diameter treatment beam. *Lasers Surg Med.* 2018;50(8):808–812.
25. Kassir R, Kolluru A, Kassir M. Intense pulsed light for the treatment of rosacea and telangiectasias. *J Cosmet Laser Ther.* 2011;13(5):216–222.
26. Taub AF. Treatment of rosacea with intense pulsed light. *J Drugs Dermatol.* 2003;2(3):254–259.
27. Lonne-Rahm S, Nordlind K, Edström DW, Ros A-M, Berg M. Laser treatment of rosacea: a pathoetiological study. *Arch Dermatol.* 2004;140(11):1345–1349.
28. Rodrigues-Braz D, Zhao M, Yesilirmak N, Aractingi S, Behar-Cohen F, Bourges JL. Cutaneous and ocular rosacea: common and specific physiopathogenic mechanisms and study models. *Mol Vis.* 2021;27:323–353.
29. Kellogg DL, Jr., Pérgola PE, Piest KL, et al. Cutaneous active vasodilation in humans is mediated by cholinergic nerve cotransmission. *Circ Res.* 1995;77(6):1222–1228.

30. Yamazaki F, Minokoshi K. Exercise training and cutaneous vasodilator function. *Jpn J Phys Fit Sports Med.* 2017;66:185–193.
31. Kellogg DL, Jr. In vivo mechanisms of cutaneous vasodilation and vasoconstriction in humans during thermoregulatory challenges. *J Appl Physiol.* 2006;100(5):1709–1718.
32. Aubdool AA, Brain SD. Neurovascular aspects of skin neurogenic inflammation. *J Investig Dermatol Symp Proc.* 2011;15(1):33–39.
33. Metzler-Wilson K, Toma K, Sammons DL, et al. Augmented supraorbital skin sympathetic nerve activity responses to symptom trigger events in rosacea patients. *J Neurophysiol.* 2015;114(3):1530–1537.
34. Moura AKA, Guedes F, Rivitti-Machado MC, Sotto MN. Inate immunity in rosacea. Langerhans cells, plasmacytoid dentritic cells, Toll-like receptors and inducible oxide nitric synthase (iNOS)expression in skin specimens: case-control study. *Arch Dermatol Res.* 2018;310(2):139–146.
35. Weinberg JB, Chen Y, Jiang N, Beasley BE, Salerno JC, Ghosh DK. Inhibition of nitric oxide synthase by cobalamins and cobinamides. *Free Radic Biol Med.* 2009;46(12):1626–1632.
36. Rochelle LG, Morana SJ, Kruszyna H, Russell MA, Wilcox DE, Smith R. Interactions between hydroxocobalamin and nitric oxide(NO): evidence for a redox reaction between NO and reduced cobalamin and reversible NO binding to oxidized cobalamin. *J Pharmacol Exp Ther.* 1995;275(1):48–52.
37. Huang Y W, Huang HP, Hsu CK, Lee JY. Hydroxocobalamin: an effective treatment for flushing and persistent erythema in rosacea. *J Clin Aesthet Dermatol.* 2022;15(6):42–45.
38. Yuraitis M, Jacob CI. Botulinum toxin for the treatment of facial flushing. *Dermatol Surg.* 2004;30(1):102–104.
39. Kranendonk SK, Ferris LK, Obagi S. Re: Botulinum toxin for the treatment of facial flushing. *Dermatol Surg.* 2005;31(4):491; author reply 492.
40. Park KY, Hyun MY, Jeong SY, Kim BJ, Kim MN, Hong CK. Botulinum toxin for the treatment of refractory erythema and flushing of rosacea. *Dermatology.* 2015;230(4):299–301.
41. Field M, Splevins A, Picaut P, et al. AbobotulinumtoxinA (Dysport®), OnabotulinumtoxinA (Botox®), and IncobotulinumtoxinA (Xeomin®) neurotoxin content and potential implications for duration of response in patients. *Toxins.* 2018;10(12).

42. Kerscher M, Wanitphakdeedecha R, Trindade de Almeida A, Maas C, Frevert J. IncobotulinumtoxinA: A highly purified and precisely manufactured Botulinum neurotoxin type A. *J Drugs Dermatol.* 2019;18(1):52–57.
43. Hong JY, Kim JH, Jin JE, Shin SH, Park KY. Practical application of novel test methods to evaluate the potency of Botulinum toxin: a comparison analysis among widely used products in Korea. *Toxins.* 2021;13(12).
44. Al-Ghamdi AS, Alghanemy N, Joharji H, Al- Qahtani D, Alghamdi H. Botulinum toxin: non cosmetic and off-label dermatological uses. *J Dermatol Surg.* 2015;19(1):1–8.
45. Go EJ, Ji J, Kim YH, Berta T, Park CK. Transient receptor potential channels and Botulinum neurotoxins in chronic pain. *Front Mol Neurosci.* 2021; 14:772719.
46. Bloom BS, Payongayong L, Mourin A, Goldberg DJ. Impact of intradermal abobotulinumtoxinA on facial erythema of rosacea. *Dermatol Surg.* 2015;41:S9–16.
47. Kim MJ, Kim JH, Cheon HI, et al. Assessment of skin physiology change and safety after intradermal injections with Botulinum toxin: a randomized, double-blind, placebo-controlled, split-face pilot study in rosacea patients with facial erythema. *Dermatol Surg.* 2019;45(9):1155–1162.
48. Friedman O, Koren A, Niv R, Mehrabi JN, Artzi O. The toxic edge-A novel treatment for refractory erythema and flushing of rosacea. *Lasers Surg Med.* 2019;51(4):325–331.
49. Al-Niaimi F, Glagoleva E, Araviiskaia E. Pulsed dye laser followed by intradermal botulinum toxin type-A in the treatment of rosacea-associated erythema and flushing. *Dermatol Ther.* 2020;33(6):e13976.
50. Fan C, Chu X, Wang L, Shi H, Li T. Botulinum toxin type A reduces TRPV1 expression in the dorsal root ganglion in rats with adjuvant- arthritis pain. *Toxicon.* 2017;133:116–122.
51. Xiao L, Cheng J, Zhuang Y, et al. Botulinum toxin type A reduces hyperalgesia and TRPV1 expression in rats with neuropathic pain. *Pain Med.* 2013;14(2):276–286.
52. Goldberg SH, Gehrman MD, Graham JH. Botulinum toxin A and B improve perfusion, increase flap survival, cause vasodilation, and prevent thrombosis: a systematic review and meta-analysis of controlled animal studies. *Hand.* 2021:1558944721994250.

53. Stone AV, Koman LA, Callahan MF, et al. The effect of Botulinum neurotoxin-A on blood flow in rats: a potential mechanism for treatment of Raynaud phenomenon. *J Hand Surg Am.* 2012;37(4):795–802.
54. Matak I, Bölcskei K, Bach-Rojecky L, Helyes Z. Mechanisms of Botulinum toxin type A action on pain. *Toxins*. 2019;11(8).
55. Aubdool AA, Brain SD. Neurovascular aspects of skin neurogenic inflammation. *J Investig Dermatol Symp Proc*. 2011;15(1):33–39.

# 3

# Treatment

## 3.1 Treatments proposed by the global ROSCO panel based on phenotypes

The 2017 ROSCO proposals for the treatment of rosacea are based on phenotypes,[1] to compensate for the inadequacy in subtype-based treatment classification in the 2002 recommendations. The 2019 global ROSCO panel reaffirmed the 2017 treatment principles.[2] Table 12 lists the treatment recommendations and common dosages for facial flushing, erythema, telangiectasia, and papulopustules.[3]

### 3.1.1 *Papulopustules*

The global ROSCO panel recommends that mild cases of papulopustules should be treated with topical ivermectin, metronidazole, and azelaic acid. Despite metronidazole being classified as an antibiotic, it has antioxidant and anti-inflammatory effects which can be used as a mechanism to treat papulopustules.[4,5] In Taiwan, only the gel-form can be prescribed. Improvements will usually be seen after 2–4 weeks, but treatment must continue for a persistent period. Topical ivermectin has shown superior efficacy compared with metronidazole in some studies. Azelaic acid inhibits the expression of cathelicidin and KLK-5, has an antioxidant and anti-inflammatory effect, and can reduce facial erythema. Significant improvements can be seen after 12–15 weeks of use. Notable potential side effects include stinging, itching, and flushing.[6] For moderate to

**Table 12.** Treatments proposed by the global ROSCO panel

| Phenotype and treatment | Dosage |
|---|---|
| Flushing | |
| β-blockers | |
| Propranolol | 20 to 40 mg 2 to 3 times per day |
| Carvedilol | 6.25 mg 2 to 3 times per day |
| α2-Adrenergic agonists | |
| Clonidine | 50 μg twice daily |
| Erythema | |
| Brimonidine 0.33% gel | 5 pea-sized amounts daily, evaluate after 6-8 weeks |
| Oxymetazoline hydrochloride 1% cream | five pea-sized amounts daily, evaluate after 6-8 weeks |
| IPL, Pulsed dye laser | Typically, 1–4 treatments at intervals of 3–4 weeks |
| Papules/pustules | |
| Mild | |
| Topical ivermectin, metronidazole, azelaic acid | Ivermectin can be used for mild, moderate, and sever cases |
| Moderate | |
| Doxycycline | 40mg or 100mg daily |
| Oral Isotretinoin | 0.25–0.3mg/kg daily |
| Telangiectasia | |
| Electrodessication | |
| IPL, pulsed dye laser, long pulsed Nd:YAG laser | Typically, 1–4 treatments at intervals of 3–4 weeks |
| Rhinophyma | |
| Inflamed | |
| Tretinoin | Once or twice daily, 8–12 weeks |
| Doxycycline | 100mg daily, 8–12 weeks |
| Oral isotretinoin | 0.25-0.3mg/kg, 3–4 months |
| Non-inflamed | |
| Surgery or ablative lasers | |

severe papulopustules, treatment with topical ivermectin is recommended.[2] Topical isotretinoin is not as effective as metronidazole and azelaic acid and is considered a second line of treatment, though attention to skin irritation is crucial. Some researchers have endorsed the effectiveness of topical benzoyl peroxide, erythromycin, and clindamycin, but the evidence in favor of such treatments is low. Pimecrolimus, a topical calcineurin inhibitor, may also be effective in the treatment of papulopustules and erythema.[7] Tacrolimus is also effective for the treatment of erythema but exhibits no significant effects in the treatment of papulopustules.[8]

Oral medications may be considered in cases of severe clinical symptoms or when there is limited response to topical medications. Oral medications include oral tetracycline, doxycycline, and minocycline, which exert their therapeutic effects through anti-inflammatory properties.[9] The macrolide antibiotics clarithromycin, azithromycin, and erythromycin are less commonly used to treat rosacea but are equally as effective for the treatment of papulopustules.[9,10] Oral isotretinoin can also be used to treat papulopustules and is effective at low doses (0.3 mg/kg each day).[11]

### 3.1.2 *Erythema*

Topical brimonidine is an α-2 adrenergic receptor agonist that has vasoconstrictive properties, but may worsen erythema.[12] Oral β-blockers decrease sympathetic activity and inhibit brown adipose tissue thermogenesis, thereby decreasing sympathetic cholinergic flushing caused by factors such as anxiety and rapid heart rates. Commonly used β-blockers to treat rosacea include propranolol and carvedilol. Furthermore, α2-adrenergic agonists also decrease sympathetic activity.[13]

### 3.1.3 *Rhinophyma*

In a retrospective study of hospital patients, 1,615 patients with rosacea included 41 (2.5%) patients with nasal rosacea. These 41 patients all (100%) had fixed erythema, whereas 17 (41.5%) patients had phymatous changes. This primarily affected middle-aged to older Caucasian men.

The lower two-thirds of the nose is the primary area of invasion.[14] The majority of our patients also have fixed erythema and only a few patients lacked fixed erythema. There are both nonsurgical and surgical treatment options for rhinophyma. Nonsurgical options include topical metronidazole, a drug which inhibits the production of reactive oxygen species and reduces skin inflammation. Another option is oral isotretinoin, a drug that inhibits the sebaceous glands and limits the production of oil and sebum. However, this medication must be discontinued in case of surgical treatment. Surgical treatments for rhinophyma include electrocauterization, freezing, and the use of ablative lasers. Dr. D K Chang et al. published a five-step technique for the treatment of rhinophyma: (1) Dermabrasion: Renewing the surface of the skin to facilitate the following steps. (2) Dermaplaning: This refers to the scraping of the affected skin without making any direct cuts, and prepares the skin's surface for the next step. (3) Debulking: Using curved scissors to trim away thickened skin. Samples will also be collected from any area that may be malignant, and sent to a laboratory for analysis. (4) Electrocautery: Damages the affected tissues. (5) Lasers: Seal wounds and create micro-contours.[15]

In the event of rhinophyma with an excess of *Demodex* mites, particularly *Demodex* folliculorum, anti-*Demodex* treatment is also

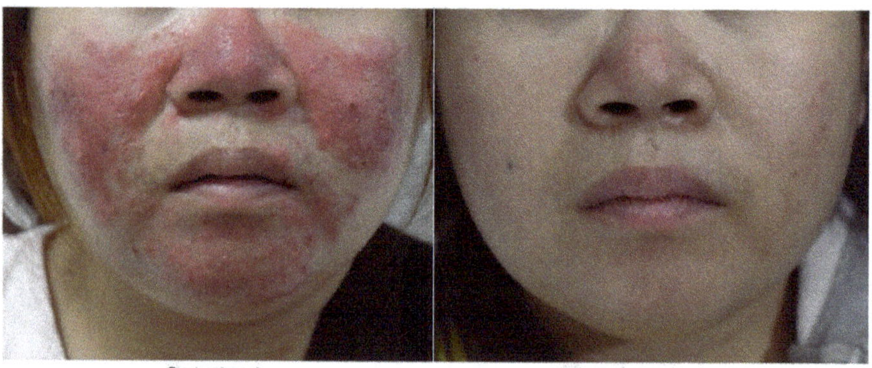


**Figure 98.** A female patient with both rosacea and rhinophyma was treated with topical ivermectin (to target *Demodex*), oral carvedilol, oral isotretinoin, pulsed dye laser treatment, and topical metronidazole. After 5.5 months, the skin was stable, and after 4 years, the patient no longer requires medication to maintain her skin condition.

recommended. However, Dr. Huang's clinical experience has shown that in some cases, topical metronidazole is still required for nasal rosacea to achieve improved results (Figure 98).

## 3.2 Pathway-level and targeted treatments: Treatment principles based on the mechanism of action on rosacea

Dr. Huang believes that there are numerous clinical questions regarding the principle of phenotypic treatment: When should monotherapy be used instead of combination therapy? Which monotherapy should be used first? After how long without seeing results should secondary treatment options be sought? What should be done in the event of a case difficult to solve? Can the medication be discontinued? What should the next steps be if relapse occurs after medication discontinuation? Here, we will introduce our own research results and clinical experiences to prioritize the treatment of rosacea via pathway-level and target treatments that are guided by the etiological and pathological mechanisms of rosacea and show that deficiencies should be targeted with phenotype-based treatments (Figure 99).

### 3.2.1 *Features of Dr. Huang's treatments for rosacea*

Identify the triggers for each individual patient before treatment:

1. Test for *Demodex* (TSM): Anti-*Demodex* medication should be used in patients with high DMD. The timing at which medication should be administered depends on the patient's condition and is described in further detail in the following section. Preventing or reducing the deterioration of rosacea caused by killing the *Demodex* is necessary.
2. Test for stress triggers: Patients with centrofacial erythema should perform arithmetic (continuous subtraction) test or an isometric hand grip test, for 2 minutes each. If the patient exhibits facial flushing, this indicates a significant skin sympathetic cholinergic vasodilation. Rosacea can be diagnosed by erythema accompanied by flushing, which can also be treated by the intradermal injection of BoNT.
3. Thermal stimulation triggers: Usually conducted via a consultation and involves testing whether the facial flushing appears under the follow-

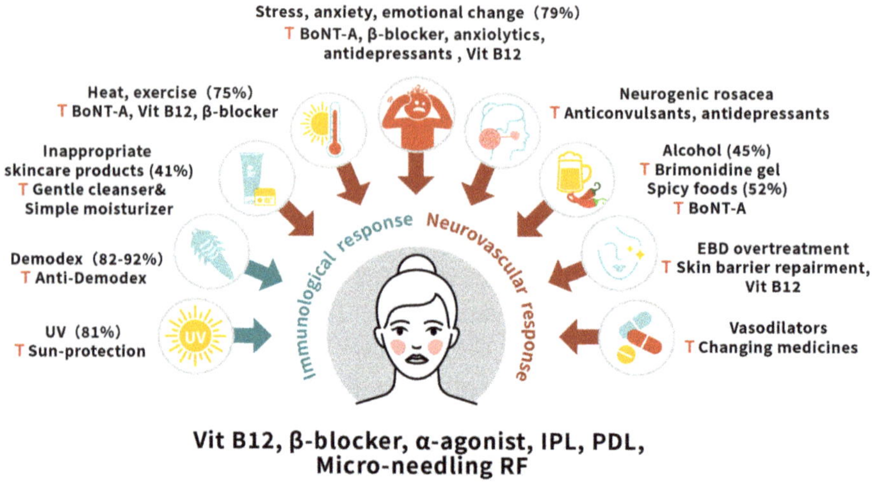


**Figure 99.** Pathway-level and targeted treatments for rosacea. There are numerous triggers for the onset of rosacea, the clearest of which must be eliminated. "T" refers to preventive or treatment methods. It is important to be aware of patients at risk of early deterioration of symptoms and take preventive measures in use of ivermectin cream.

References: Ratio based on that of the National Rosacea Society, United States of America Website information and published research *Australas J Dermatol*. 2017;58(2):e26–e30 and *J Eur Acad Dermatol Venereol*. 2020;34(7):e343–e345.

ing activities: exercise, using a blow dryer, taking a hot shower, cooking and frying food (such as fish), and after 10 minutes of intense exercise. Thermal stimulation can be categorized into systemic thermal stimulation, which involves an increase in core body temperature, and localized thermal stimulation. The flushing mechanism of systemic thermal stimulation is a sympathetic response. Non-nociceptive localized thermal stimulation can be divided into two stages of response: the first wave of flushing is induced by the antidromic release of vasoactive peptides via the activation of TRPV-1 in the sensory nerves; the second wave occurs as the temperature continues to rise, which is a high-intensity and persistent flushing associated with NO. Skin sympathetic cholinergic flushing and afferent sensory flushing can be treated via intradermal injection of BoNT, whereas persistent flushing can be treated using the NO scavenger hydroxocobalamin.

4. Drug history: Patients currently taking prescribed medication must ensure they are not taking any medications which may induce vasodi-

lation and facial flushing, particularly calcium channel blocker amlodipine, which is one of the most common causes of facial flushing among patients with hypertension in our clinic.

5. Neurogenic rosacea: In patients with severe erythema encroaching the facial perimeters, including the outer cheeks, upper eyelids, ears, and close to the neck, along with burning and stinging sensations, it may be associated with neuropsychiatric or rheumatoid comorbidity.
6. Testing the role of NO: Changes in facial flushing after 40 minutes of outpatient hydroxocobalamin testing.

For comparison, Tables 13 and 14 present Dr Huang's treatments, the global treatment consensus, and the most recent treatment consensus or guidelines from various countries.[1,2,16–18]

### 3.2.2 *Mechanism of action of rosacea and etiological and pathological pathway targets*

In the treatment of rosacea, we have developed pathway-level and targeted treatments based on phenotypes.[9,17–22] Summarizing both the existing literature and our own research, the functions and mechanisms of topical, systemic, and injectable medications, as well as energy-based devices for the treatment of rosacea are detailed in Table 15. Pathway-level and targeted treatments are shown in Table 16. Etiological and pathological pathway targets and treatment options are shown in Figure 100.

*Demodex* and UV rays trigger an innate immune response.[9] These two pathways can be halted at the source by both protecting oneself against the UV rays of the sun and taking anti-*Demodex* strategies, including medication such as topical ivermectin[23,24] and permethrin,[25] in the event that a high DMD is determined. Ivermectin binds with GABA or glutamate-gated chloride channels, and has been found to paralyze motor neurons and pharyngeal muscles in invertebrates (nematodes). This results in paralysis or death due to starvation.[26]

Ivermectin cream should be administered while a preventive treatment is formulated based on the patient's condition to avoid the worsening of rosacea (Table 17).[24,27] Oral isotretinoin inhibits monocyte TLR-2 expression and subsequent inflammatory cytokine responses.[11] Carvedilol inhibits the TLR2/KLK5/cathelicidin response pathway in macrophages.[28]

**Table 13.** Treatment of transient erythema, persistent erythema, and telangiectasia in patients with rosacea

| Cutaneous features | Hui-Peng Huang | 2017/2019 Global rosacea consensus (ROSCO) | 2020 Brazilian consensus | 2021 British guideline | 2019 Spanish Consensus |
|---|---|---|---|---|---|
| Transient erythema | NO scavenger (hydroxocobalamin β-blockers) Propranolol Carvedilol<br>Intradermal botulinum toxin A | β-blockers Propranolol Carvedilol<br>α2-A drenergic agonists Clonidine | Soothing masks with chamomile, feverfew, green tea etc.<br>Intradermal botulinum toxin A | Oral propranolol<br>Topical brimonidine | 1 st-line therapy Topical brimonidine Topical brimonidine + vascular laser therapy or IPL<br>2nd-line therapy<br>Oral β-blockers (off-label) |
| Persistent erythema | NO scavenger (hydroxocobalamin)<br>Topical ivermectin if *Demodex* density is high<br>Intradermal botulinum toxin A<br>PDL or IPL (for patients with a low *Demodex* density and CEA<3) | Brimonidine (0.33% gel)<br>(α-A drenergic agonists)<br>Oxymetazoline hydrochloride (1% cream) (selective α1 and partial α2 adrenergic agonist)<br>IPL, PDL | Topical α-adrenergic agonist (brimonidine)<br>Pulsed light or laser<br>Intradermal botulinum toxin A | PDL, Nd:YAG laser or IPL<br>Topical brimonidine | 1st-line therapy PDL, IPL Topical brimonidine PDL or IPL + topical brimonidine<br>2nd-line therapy Other vascular laser therapies Oral β-blockers (off label) |
| Telangiectasia | PDL, IPL, Non-insulated micro-needle pulsed radiofrequency | Electrodesiccation IPL, PDL, Nd:YAG laser, or other lasers | Electrocauterization Laser or pulsed light | | 1st-line therapy<br>PDL, IPL<br>2nd-line therapy Electrodesiccation |

Note: CEA, Clinician's Erythema Assessment; IPL, intense pulsed light, PDL, pulsed dye laser.

**Table 14.** Treatment of inflammatory papules and pustules in patients with rosacea

| Hui-Peng Huang | 2017/2019 global rosacea consensus (ROSCO) | 2020 Brazilian consensus | 2021 British guideline |
|---|---|---|---|
| High *Demodex* density<br>Topical ivermectin with proper combination (doxycycline, 1st week-low potency steroid) to prevent flare<br>Low *Demodex* density<br>1st line<br>Local: metronidazole or azelaic acid<br>Systemic: doxycycline<br>2nd line<br>Oral isotretinoin | Mild<br>Local: azelaic acid, ivermectin, metronidazole;<br>Systemic: doxycycline<br>Moderate<br>Local: azelaic acid, ivermectin, metronidazole;<br>Systemic: doxycycline<br>Severe<br>Local: ivermectin;<br>Systemic: doxycycline, isotretinoin | Mild/moderate<br>Local: azelaic acid, ivermectin, metronidazole; Systemic: doxycycline<br>Other options: tetracycline, azithromycin, limecycline, minocycline, topical alpha-agonists, sulfacetamide, calcineurin inhibitors, topical retinoids<br>Severe<br>Topical ivermectin<br>Oral doxycycline (40 mg/day)<br>Oral isotretinoin (0.25–0.3 mg/kg/day) | Offer<br>Topical ivermectin, metronidazole or azelaic acid an oral antibiotic (severe cases)<br>Consider minocycline foam<br>Consider low-dose isotretinoin, e.g., 0.25 mg $kg^{-1}$ (persistent and severe cases; when a course of oral antibiotics has failed, or to avoid prescribing long-term antibiotic) |

**Table 15.** Effects and mechanism of medications and photoelectric apparatus used in the treatment of rosacea

| | Effects | Mechanism | Notes |
|---|---|---|---|
| Ivermectin (topical) | Antiparasite, Anti-inflammation | Binds GABA- or Glutamate-gated chloride ion channel, inhibits NF-κβ pathway, and decreases the production of proinflammatory cytokines | Reduction of mites helps improve erythema and papulopustules |
| Azelaic acid (topical) | Anti-inflammation | Reduces ROS, inhibits UVB-induced upregulation of proinflammatory cytokines, inhibits cathelicidin, and KLK5 activity | Literature recommends 15% cream, though in Taiwan only the 20% cream is available, which is more irritating. |
| Metronidazole (topical) | Anti-inflammatory or immunosuppressive actions | Unclear, reduces and inactivates ROS | In Taiwan, only the gel is approved. |
| Brimonidine (topical) | α2-adrenergic receptor agonists | Vasoconstriction of cutaneous arterioles | Paradoxical erythema reaction and allergic contact dermatitis |
| Tacrolimus, pimecrolimus (topical) | Anti-inflammatory properties of calcineurin inhibitors | Blocks T cell activation and thereby reduce the further release of proinflammatory cytokines | May induce rosacea-like dermatitis |
| Tranexamic acid soaking | Restore barrier function Vasoconstriction | Inhibits protease- activated receptor-2, suppresses plasmin-induced angiogenesis, and suppresses endothelin-1 | Reduce erythema |
| Doxycycline, minocycline | Anti-inflammation | Inhibits MMPs, indirectly inhibits KLK- 5, and inhibits the NO synthase | The subantimicrobial dose is preferred |
| Isotretinoin (Oral) | Downregulate TLR-2 expression | Downregulates TLR-2 expression and promotes atrophy of sebaceous glands | |

| | | | |
|---|---|---|---|
| Propranolol | Non-selective (β1,2-) adrenergic receptor antagonist, anti-anxiety | Vasoconstriction | Side effect: Bradycardia and hypotension |
| Carvedilol | Non-specific β-adrenergic receptor antagonist, anti-oxidant, alleviate the inflammatory reaction, anxiolytic effect | Vasoconstriction of dermal vasculatures, inhibit the TLR2/KLK5/cathelicidin pathway in macrophages | Side effect: Bradycardia and hypotension. A third-generation β-blocker should be a first-choice β-blocker |
| Gabapentin or pregabalin | Anti-epileptic activity. | Binding alpha2-delta Type 1 protein, reduced neurotransmitter releasing such as substance P, CGRP, noradrenaline and acetylcholine | Treatment for neurogenic rosacea |
| Hydroxocobalamin | NO scavenger | Inhibit NO synthases, reversible binding to NO. | |
| Botulinum toxin A | Decrease sympathetic flushing triggered by an increase in core body temperature | Cleave SNAP25 protein. Blockage of skin sympathetic cholinergic co-transmitters. Indirect inhibition of mast cell degranulation. | |
| Hydroxychloroquine | Inhibits the infiltration and activation of mast cells | Inhibiting KCa3.1-mediated Ca2+ signaling | |
| Pulsed dye laser | Selective photothermolysis | Decrease in the immunoreactivity of substance P-positive nerve fibers, remodeling of dermal collagen and coagulation of vascular structure | |
| Intense pulsed light | Selective photothermolysis | Remodeling of dermal collagen and vascular structure | |

KLK-5, KLK5 kallikrein related peptidase 5; NO, nitric oxide; ROS, reactive oxygen species; TLR-2, Toll-like receptor-2.

**Table 16.** Pathway-level or targeted treatment for rosacea

| Trigger factor | Test | Phenotype of rosacea | Treatment |
|---|---|---|---|
| *Demodex* | TSM, SNS, SSSB (1+2), RCM | Papule/pustules Persistent erythema | Topical ivermectin |
| Anxiety | | Persistent/transient erythema | β-adrenergic blockers |
| Stress, whole body heat | Mental arithmetic test or isometric handgrip provokes flushing | Persistent/transient erythema | Botulinum toxin A |
| Prolonged local heat, prolonged exercise | | Persistent/transient erythema | Hydroxocobalamin |

TSM, thumbnail-squeezing method; SNS, superficial needle-scraping; SSSB (1 + 2), two consecutive standardized skin surface biopsies; RCM, reflectance confocal microscope.

The anti-inflammatory response of azelaic acid may be caused by the inhibition of KLK-5, the reduction of reactive oxygen species (ROS), and the inhibition of UVB-induced upregulation of proinflammatory cytokines.[6,9] Other drugs that inhibit proinflammatory cytokines and chemokines include doxycycline, ivermectin, and metronidazole, as well as calcineurin inhibitors. The anti-inflammatory effects of doxycycline are the result of the indirect inhibition of KLK-5 and the inhibition of MMPs. It also functions as an inhibitor of NOS.[9] Ivermectin inhibits epidermal KLK-5 gene expression[29] and the NF-κβ pathway for the production of proinflammatory cytokines.[30] The mechanism of action for metronidazole's anti-inflammatory and immunosuppressive effects is not known but may be linked to the reduction in ROS.[4,5] Calcineurin inhibitors block T cell activation, further reducing proinflammatory cytokine production.[9]

In terms of neurovascular dysregulatory responses, there are two sets of sympathetic nerve branches that correspond with vascular tone in human skin, the first of which is the adrenergic vasoconstrictor system and the second is the cholinergic active vasodilator system. The latter system is not present in hairless skin, including the palms, soles of the feet, and the lips. The former system maintains appropriate vasoconstrictor tone at standard

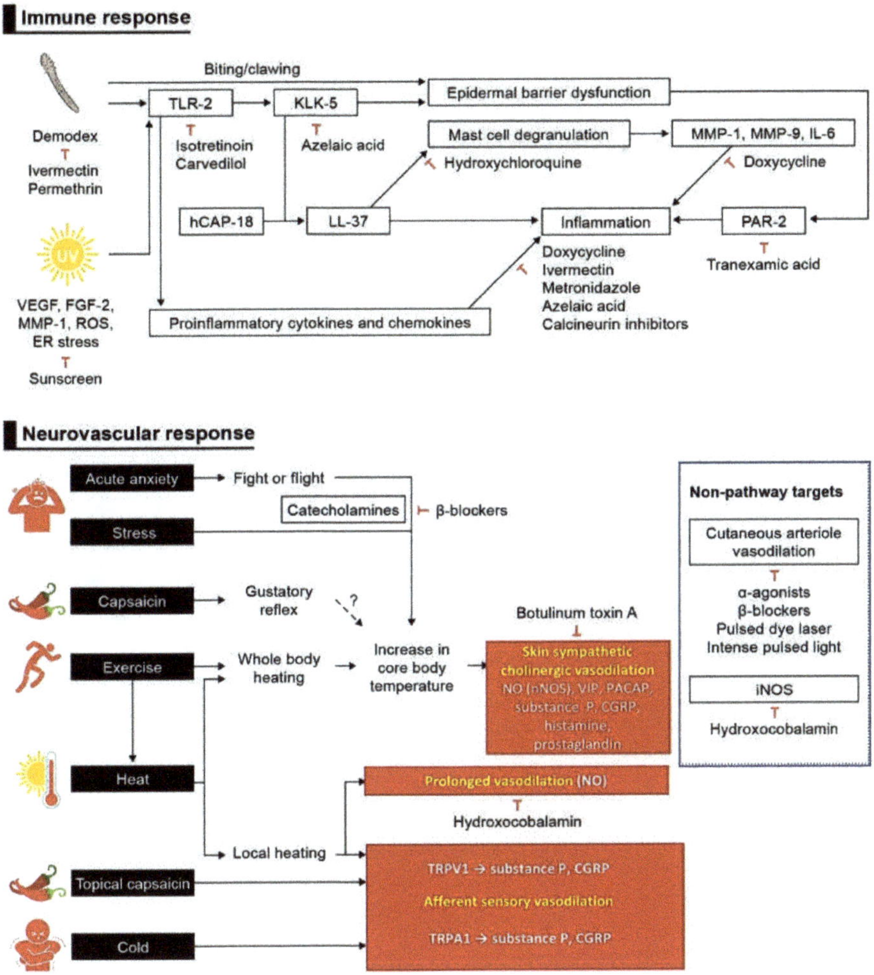


**Figure 100.** Topical medication, systemic medication, injectable medication, and photoelectric laser treatments for rosacea with etiological and pathological pathway targets. *Demodex* and UV rays trigger an innate immune response. These two pathways can be halted at the source by both protecting oneself against the UV rays of the sun and taking acaricidal medication in the event that a high *Demodex* density is discovered. Mite treatment should be administered while a preventive treatment is formulated based on the patient's condition to avoid the exacerbation of rosacea. In terms of the neurovascular dysregulatory response, triggers cannot be completely eliminated, but some targets along the pathways can be controlled. For example, a rise in systemic core temperature and stress (psychological or physiological) induces skin sympathetic cholinergic vasodilation, which can be inhibited using BoNT treatments. Persistent facial flushing caused by high facial temperature (resulting from long hot showers or persistent blow drying of the hair) and

**Table 17.** Incidence of early exacerbation, possible mechanism of action, and recommended preventive measures associated with the treatment using topical ivermectin.

| | Incidence | Possible mechanism of action | Recommendations |
|---|---|---|---|
| Steroid use, followed by sudden discontinuance | 100% | 1. Steroid rebound 2. Large accumulation of dead mites in the hair follicles | Extend use of steroids for 1–2 weeks |
| Papules | 75% | Unknown | First target inflammation, then use anti-*Demodex* treatment |
| Papulopustules | 38% | Large accumulation of dead mites in the hair follicles | Use weak localized steroid for 1 week |
| Ivermectin cream only | 24% | Large accumulation of dead mites in hair follicles | low-potency topical steroids for 1 week with carvedilol |
| Ivermectin cream with carvedilol | 5.4% | Large accumulation of dead mites in hair follicles | Use weak localized steroid for 1 week |
| Ivermectin cream Use weak localized steroid for 1 week | 1.4% | 1. Steroids not strong enough 2. No actual use of steroids 3. Large accumulation of dead mites in hair follicles | Prophylactic steroid use for 1 week |

**Figure 100. (*Continued*)** intense exercise may be reduced or prevented using hydroxocobalamin. By inhibiting the thermal stimulation and the significant facial flushing mechanism associated with exercise, patients with rosacea are able to exercise without prominent flushing. Acute stress and anxiety induce the fight or flight response, and β-blockers such as carvedilol and propranolol inhibit the sympathetic tone, and thermogenic effect of brown adipose tissue. In terms of nonpathway targets, α2-adrenergic agonists (clonidine and topical brimonidine), nonselective α adrenergic agonist (oxymetazoline), and β-blockers constrict cutaneous arterioles, and pulsed dye lasers and intense pulsed light cause selective hemoglobin heat absorption which coagulates blood vessels. Patients with rosacea experience higher levels of iNOS than normal individuals, and hydroxocobalamin can inhibit iNOS. "T" represents forms of prevention or treatment.

References: Modified from Rosacea: Molecular mechanisms and management of a chronic cutaneous inflammatory condition. *Int J Mol Sci*. 2016;17(9).

temperatures and at rest, becoming more active as the skin and core temperature drop. An increase in the core temperature of the body activates the cholinergic active vasodilator system, causing a significant increase in blood flow to the skin.[31] Acute stress induces cutaneous vasoconstriction and peripheral blood flow reduction, along with β3-adrenergic receptor upregulation in brown adipose tissue, leading to an increase in core temperature.[32,33] In addition, 80% of the energy released by the muscles during exercise is converted into heat. This raises the core body temperature, which further triggers the skin sympathetic cholinergic vasodilator response.[19,31] Rosacea triggers (including heat, stress, and anxiety) cannot be completely eliminated, but some targets along the pathways can be controlled. By inhibiting the thermal stimulation and facial flushing mechanism associated with exercise, patients with rosacea are able to exercise with minimal issues. Additionally, skin sympathetic cholinergic flushing caused by acute stress and increases in core temperature can be inhibited using BoNT-A.[19] Clinically, Dr. Huang uses the arithmetic and isometric grip tests to assess whether a patient experiences flushing, whether BoNT-A treatment will be effective, and whether repeated treatments will be necessary. Persistent facial flushing caused by high facial temperature (resulting from long hot showers, blow drying hair, and frying fish) and persistent exercise may be related to intravascular NO.[20]

Patients with rosacea experience higher levels of iNOS than normal individuals,[34] and hydroxocobalamin is able to inhibit all three types of NOS, including iNOS, in addition to binding with NO to form a ligand.[35] Therefore, hydroxocobalamin can be used to ease erythema or prevent prolonged facial flushing.[21] However, the use of hydroxocobalamin in patients with neurogenic rosacea may worsen erythema and facial flushing, and its mechanism leading to worsening may be related to mast cell. NO is a regulator of mast cell activation and mast cell-mediated inflammation.[36] Inhibition of NO by hydroxocobalamin may lead to a decrease in inhibition of the activation and degranulation of mast cells. Acute stress and anxiety trigger the fight or flight response, which involves the activation of the sympathetic nervous system and the secretion of catecholamines and cortisol into the bloodstream via pituitary to adrenal glands, resulting in vasodilation of the heart, brain, and skeletal muscles. This is accompanied by vasoconstriction in the skin and digestive system and a rise in core body temperature, which induces cutaneous vasodilation. β-blockers such as carvedilol and propranolol have anxiolytic effects, inhibit vasodilation, inhibit the thermogenetic effects of noradrenaline, and decrease the sympathetic activity.[33] The mechanism by which tranexamic acid alleviates erythema is likely via its inhibition of protease-activated receptor-2 (PAR-2), accompanied by the repairment of the epidermal barrier, suppression of endothelin-1 leading to vasoconstriction, and inhibition of plasmin-induced angiogenesis.[37–40]

## 3.3 Treatment myths debunked

### 3.3.1 *What are the benefits of anti-Demodex treatment for papulopustular rosacea?*

For those with PPR and a high DMD, the benefits of anti-*Demodex* treatment are as follows: (1) High success rate in treating pustules, (2) no need for maintenance treatment, and (3) long-term elimination of papulopustules. Physicians who disapprove the anti-*Demodex* treatment may argue that the difference between the success rates of ivermectin 1% cream and metronidazole 0.75% cream is only 10%, and the disease-free period is only 1 month longer.[40,41] In reality, the treatment success rate and rosacea remission period can be improved through increased dosages, longer treatment periods, prevention or immediate treatment of rosacea prior to flare-up, and treating papules prior to administering anti-*Demodex* treatments. The remission period can be prolonged by four-fold when the number of *Demodex* mites are reduced to that in normal individuals (Figure 25). In some patients, scattered superficial and tiny pustules will remain after the *Demodex* mites are removed. In such cases, fusidic acid treatment can be administered. When the *Demodex* mites are removed and the pustules associated with PPR fade, the rosacea shall be classified as ETR. The erythema will also reduce in severity by one or two grades. Most of pustular erythema is seemingly easy to treat. However, there are always exceptions. Doctors who disapprove the anti-*Demodex* treatment for PPR may state that taking isotretinoin is also effective, which is true; however, what happens when a patient stops taking isotretinoin? Pustules will develop once isotretinoin treatment is discontinued.

### 3.3.2 *What are the diseases, if in comorbidity with pustular rosacea, will affect the outcome of treatment for pustules?*

There are four types of common diseases which affect the outcome of treatment for pustular rosacea: (1) *H. pylori* infection. Patients with rosacea and *H. pylori* infection will need to combine rosacea treatment with the treatment for *H. pylori* infection to avoid unfavorable results in the treatment of pustules. (2) EPF often leads to an increased number of papules than pustules; thus, removal of *Demodex* mites and treatment of rosacea will only result in partial effects. These treatments should be combined with indomethacin to achieve successful results. (3) Perioral dermatitis is considered prior to treatment and should be administered with azithromycin or clarithromycin for the most significant results. If the aforementioned three comorbidities are not treated alongside rosacea, the results will be only partially effective. (4) Scattered small and superficial pustules can occur in two circumstances: The first one is that after the fading of pustules associated with demodicosis, in which the pustules are unrelated to *Demodex* and can develop after a period of time. The second circumstance is that after anti-*Demodex* treatment removes the *Demodex* mites, the pustules are only reduced and not completely disappeared. These scattered superficial pustules require a weak topical steroid or fusidic acid treatment.

### 3.3.3 *How to administer topical ivermectin properly?*

#### 3.3.3.1 *Screening patients*

Approximately 92% of patients with PPR have a high DMD, meaning that only 8% of patients have densities lower than the diagnostic criteria.[42] When topical ivermectin is used for the treatment, the clinical treatment outcome should be improved substantially, provided that patients with standard DMD are excluded. Screening for *Demodex* prior to treatment is therefore a vital step. The advantages and disadvantages of all screening methods are detailed in Table 4.

#### 3.3.3.2 *Single dose*

The original manufacturer instructions recommend that five areas of the face, including the forehead, nose, chin, and cheeks, are administered with a pea-sized dose of medicine once a day. In 2015, the original manufacturer published findings stating that 83% of patients with PPR experienced complete or almost complete clearance of papulopustules after treatment.[43] In a long-term follow-up study, 50% of patients remained free from the recurrence of papulopustules for 115 days.[41] Our research showed that the efficacy of topical ivermectin was associated with the dosage used; an incremental increase in efficacy was observed when five pea-sized doses per day, two finger tip unit doses daily, and two finger tip unit doses twice a day (Figure 59) were compared, where two finger tip unit doses are equivalent to 1 g.

#### 3.3.3.3 *Treatment duration*

The duration of treatment for topical ivermectin is associated with the therapeutic efficacy of papulopustules. Taieb et al. demonstrated a 75.7% and 83% reduction in papulopustules at weeks 12 and 16 of treatment, respectively.[42] In our statistics, among 35 patients with PPR, 24 patients were treated successfully and achieved either complete or almost complete clearance of papulopustules. In addition, 11 patients showed clinical improvement but not to the point of success. We found no statistical difference in the total dosages of topical ivermectin provided to these two groups of patients but found significant differences in the duration of treatment, with a duration of 8.0 ± 3.8 weeks (4–16 weeks) in the successful group and a duration of 4.8 ± 1.9 weeks (2–8 weeks) in the clinical improvement group. Therefore, even if the treatment dosage is identical, the extension of the treatment duration can improve the treatment efficacy of papulopustules (Figures 51 and 52).

#### 3.3.3.4 *Demodex mite density at drug discontinuation*

The lower the final DMD, the efficacy of treatment increases. The final DMD in the aforementioned successful treatment group was 7.5 ± 2.2

mites/cm$^2$, and the density is below the diagnostic threshold. The final average DMD in the treatment-induced improvement group was 23.4 ± 10.7 mites/cm$^2$, and the density is approximately twice the diagnostic cutoff value. Therefore, we concluded that the extension of the treatment duration can help reduce *Demodex* mites, even without a total dosage increase (Figures 51 and 52). We tracked all patients with rosacea treated with topical ivermectin in 2017, and they had high DMD. A 4.5-year follow-up study found 63 relapse patients having a complete record of DMD, with a final average DMD of 8.1 ± 1.95 mites/cm$^2$ for an average of 20 ± 10.3 months between the first days of two consecutive courses of treatment and a median of 18 months. The results of these two studies show that a normal DMD value after treatment results in a better healing efficacy and a longer duration without relapse (Figure 25).

#### 3.3.3.5 *Demodex density monitoring during treatment*

During the treatment period, it is important to monitor changes in clinical symptoms and DMD. We used the TSM to collect data from 23 patients treated with ivermectin cream, and we plotted a curve of time against DMD based on these data. This enables us to refer to patients undergoing treatment against the curve to understand whether or not they are aligned with average density. When the patients deviate too far from the curve (Figure 101), they must be carefully evaluated to assess their single dosage, cream application time, drug resistance, and combined treatment with oral isotretinoin or second-line anti-*Demodex* treatment.

### 3.3.4 *Is there any comparable clinical benefit from the persistent use of high-dose ivermectin cream?*

With a dosage of 1 g/day, there will be a significant decline in *Demodex* for the first 1–2 weeks, after which the decline curve will flatten (Figure 101). The first 2 weeks are similar to a 100-m sprint, whereas the following weeks are similar to a long-distance race. Theoretically, after 1 month, the dosage could be reduced to 0.5 g/day, and the extension of the treatment duration is reasonable.

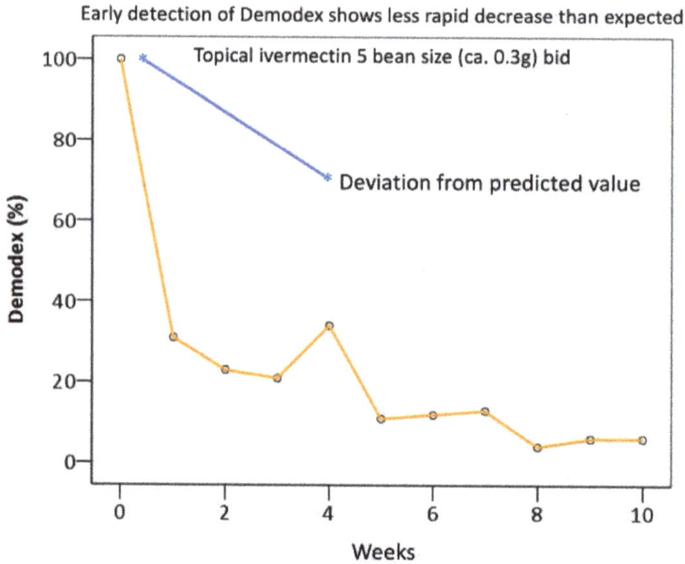


**Figure 101.** Monitoring *Demodex* density during treatment with ivermectin 1% cream allows for an assessment of density deviation from the average *Demodex* density reduction curve. When the deviation is too high (represented by the blue curve), the cause must be carefully investigated. The orange line represents the average *Demodex* density reduction.

### 3.3.5 *Are there any disadvantages to using high-dose topical ivermectin?*

Indeed, the dosage of ivermectin cream influences its anti-*Demodex* efficacy, clinical efficacy, and treatment duration. In Taieb et al.'s study of using five pea-sized doses of ivermectin per day, the only side effects recorded were skin irritation, itchiness, and burning sensation, without papulopustules or erythema flare-up.[43] However, when we began using ivermectin cream, we found that just one pea-sized dose of the cream per day for three continuous days triggered papulopustules or erythema flare.

Among the patients administered with approximately 0.3-g topical ivermectin twice per day, we found that clinical deterioration of symptoms almost always occurred in the first week. Therefore, we observed changes in DMD on the face at 8 h, 12 h, 24 h, 2 days, 3 days, 4 days, 5 days, 6 days, 7 days, and 10 days of the application of ivermectin cream. We used the TSM to observe the form of the *Demodex* mites and found that dead *Demodex* mites began to appear at the 12-h mark. Many dead *Demodex* mites could be seen within 1 week, and clumps of dead *Demodex* mites were even found in the solid sebum of the hair follicles. After the first week, it became much more difficult to locate dead *Demodex* mites. Only one or two dead *Demodex* mites were scattered sparsely. This leads us to suspect that the short-term deterioration of symptoms in the first week is probably caused by an immune response to the accumulation of dead *Demodex* mites in hair follicles, which in turn worsens papulopustules. The use of a high-dose ivermectin cream can remove *Demodex* mites more quickly, but it also has the potential to increase the chance of a flare-up. Nevertheless, we have effective methods to prevent such flare-ups.[27]

### 3.3.6 *What are the methods for preventing symptom exacerbation caused by topical ivermectin treatment in the early stages?*

Anti-*Demodex* treatment can be used to prevent early exacerbation, and special attention should be paid to patients at high risk of early exacerbation. Such patients include those with PPR, with prior use of topical steroids, with prior exacerbation caused by ivermectin cream, and treated with ivermectin cream alone. The incidence of early exacerbation, the possible mechanism of action, and the recommended preventive measures are detailed in Table 17.

#### 3.3.6.1 *Check the patient's previous and current use of topical steroids before treatment*

Patients with high DMD, who have already been treated with topical steroids for a certain duration, must take care when subjected to anti-*Demodex* treatment because of topical steroids having suppressed their immune response. When steroid treatment is halted suddenly, the original papulopustules may rebound. Moreover, in the first week of using topical ivermectin, a large number of dead *Demodex* mites will accumulate in the hair follicles, leading to a higher likelihood of short-term exacerbation of papulopustules and erythema (Figure 102) with an incidence rate of

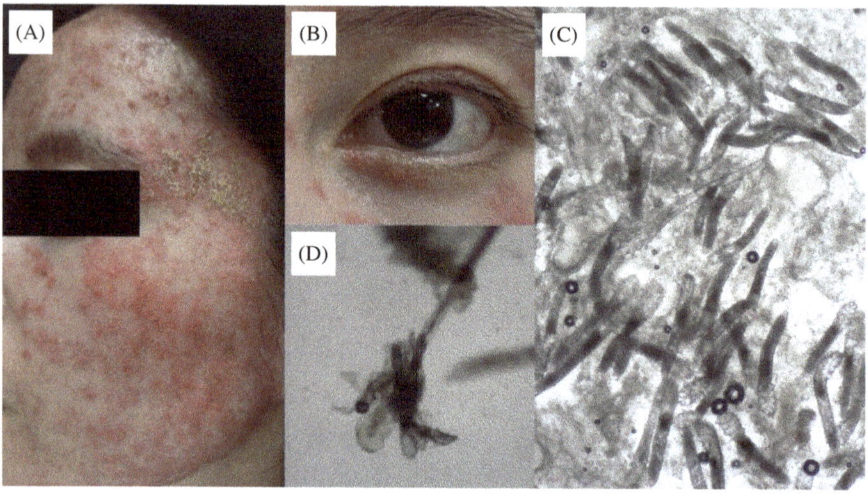


**Figure 102.** A 31-year-old woman complained that 2 weeks earlier she had experienced the sudden onset of (A) a large area of papulopustules and yellowish crust on the face and (B) yellowish crust and pustules on the eyelids. After the patient's medical history was checked, the patient had been receiving treatment for acne vulgaris and rosacea for the past 4 years, had been using steroids for the past 6 months, and began to have small papules in the past month. Two weeks ago, after forgetting to take her steroids, she experienced a breakout of papulopustules the following day. (C) Through the thumbnail-squeezing method, we detected 528 mites/cm$^2$ on her face and (D) 13 mites on four eyelashes.

almost 100%. The conservative treatment method involves the continued use of steroids for 1 week.

If the patient experiences steroid-induced skin atrophy, telangiectasia, and sensitive, flaky skin, the patient should switch to tacrolimus 0.1% ointment in the second week. Because it can cause side effects of burning and itching, a small amount of Protopic and a small amount of topical ivermectin are recommended. The dosage should be increased gradually to the size of two finger tip units to avoid the sudden accumulation of excessive dead *Demodex* mites in the hair follicles, which increases the risk of exacerbation.

### 3.3.6.2 *Weak steroids for prevention*

Patients with rosacea taking high-dose topical ivermectin are expected to show rapid clinical improvements along with a longer disease remission time. However, the patients are also exposed to a higher risk of their rosacea being exacerbated in the first week of treatment. There is strong evidence to suggest that when a large number of dead *Demodex* mites accumulate within hair follicles, their exoskeletal chitin and microorganisms within the *Demodex* mites trigger an innate immune response and an adaptive immune response. Fortunately, such responses can be treated or prevented using topical steroids. Therefore, during the first week of treatment with ivermectin cream, we can prescribe a weak steroid in advance, applying dots of cream to existing pustules, pustules caused by dead *Demodex* mites, or to new and exacerbated erythema. From July to December 2020, we treated 178 patients with rosacea concurrent with *Demodex* overgrowth. They were prescribed with two finger tip units per day and a weak steroid (clobetasone butyrate) in the first week. The results showed that only two patients out of 146 (1.4%) experienced early exacerbation in the first week.[27] The negative reaction in these two patients can be traced back to the fact that when the first pustule became exacerbated, they were afraid to use the recommended topical steroid, leading to more papulopustules developing the following day.

### 3.3.6.3 *Combination with carvedilol or other anti-inflammatory medicines*

Topical ivermectin in combination with oral carvedilol can effectively alleviate early exacerbation. In our clinical study, 24% of patients with rosacea who solely used topical ivermectin experienced exacerbation in the first week; however, among 22 patients who used ivermectin cream in combination with oral carvedilol, only 4.5% of them experienced early exacerbation.[24] A possible explanation for such a difference is that carvedilol inhibits the innate immunity (TLR-2) of macrophages, as reported in a 2021 study by Zhang.[28] Other anti-inflammatory drugs are also likely to reduce early exacerbation of symptoms, particularly in purely papular rosacea, wherein doxycycline plays a very important role. However, we have a limited number of cases and have not made any statistical analyses based on these drugs. Those with purely papular rosacea receiving ivermectin cream treatment have an exacerbation incidence rate of 75% and are recommended to take oral doxycycline and topical metronidazole to reduce inflammation and remove *Demodex* mites in a safer and appropriate manner.

#### 3.3.6.4 *Special face washing methods to remove dead Demodex*

Early exacerbation is strongly associated with the accumulation of dead *Demodex* mites in the hair follicles. Therefore, in the first week of treatment, a foaming cleanser should be used to rub and pinch the skin rapidly, which will emulsify and soften the sebum and accumulated dead *Demodex* mites within the hair follicles. Because of the potential for skin irritation, individuals with papulopustules, inflammation, and neurogenic rosacea are not recommended to rub and pinch the skin. In other cases, patients have reported that washing their face in such a way feels good, and leaves the skin feeling cleansed. We have named this the "explosive face washing method."

### 3.3.7 *How to determine a suitable dosage of topical ivermectin for patients?*

The key point we have talked about so far is that topical ivermectin is only used when there is *Demodex* overgrowth. The way to determine if there are too many mites is by testing the density of mites. Patients with rosacea with excessive *Demodex* can use five pea-sized doses a day, 1 g (the size of two finger tip units) a day, or 2 g a day. In what circumstances would we want to use a low dosage? And in what circumstances would we want to use a high dosage? And finally, in what circumstances would no difference be made between a low or high dosage?

First, in the case of a patient with mild to moderate erythema and enlarged pores, both a low or high dosage is acceptable. The only difference lies in the time taken for the treatment to stabilize, and the duration in which it will remain stable in the future. In the event of a patient wanting to become pregnant, her symptoms should be treated slowly with drugs such as permethrin or topical ivermectin should be used to stabilize rosacea and normalize the *Demodex* density within 2–4 weeks. To complete a course of treatment in such a short duration, a high dosage of 2 g once a day will be suitable to achieve such a target. This also implies that complementary preventive measures against early exacerbation must also be fully implemented.

In what circumstances, then, would a high dose be unsuitable? In the event that the patient's rosacea primarily manifests as papules, even five pea-sized doses will be excessive to begin with. Instead, two pea-sized doses are given to observe whether the patient experiences any exacerbation of symptoms. Typically, these patients are apprehensive of experiencing a granulomatous reaction; thus, a low dose of topical ivermectin combined with anti-inflammatory drugs, particularly doxycycline, is the safest method of treatment. A very small dose of topical ivermectin should also be used for patients with irritation, as these cases may develop blisters, exacerbated erythema, or new areas of erythema. There is an even greater need to pay special attention to those who experience delayed onset of such symptoms. A patch test on the skin of the forearm can be used to assess whether a patient is allergic to ivermectin.

### 3.3.8 *Although ivermectin is for the eradication of mites, why does the treatment not work on my pustules?*

This is a common question online from confused individuals wondering why, when they have clearly used four tubes of ivermectin cream, have their pustules not been cleared? In fact, pustules on the face are not solely caused by rosacea, nor is rosacea only caused by the presence of *Demodex*. Thus, a detailed assessment, appropriate diagnosis, and DMD assessment are necessary both before and at the end of treatment. Not assessing *Demodex* does not provide a clear picture and will lead to poor results or the rapid recurrence of symptoms. In our outpatient clinic, we administer anti-*Demodex* treatments only under the excessively high pretreatment DMD and will stop administering such drugs when the number of *Demodex* mites have dropped to the normal post-treatment value. We track patient progress for 4.5 years. Comparing the duration when patients have no papulopustules, the median duration for patients assessed for DMD and combined with comprehensive treatment is 18 months, whereas in the previous reports, the median duration for patients who have not undergone assessment but have taken 16 weeks of topical ivermectin treatment is 115 days (3.8 months),[41] where the latter is four-fold lower than the former in terms of the median duration. Comparing these two figures, it is clear that DMD assessment is crucial.

Many diseases of the face must be differentiated from demodicosis, and there are some which may be present alongside *Demodex*, meaning that *Demodex* assessment and conclusive diagnosis are closely linked. For those with PPR, is *Demodex* removal enough to resolve their condition? Following are the conditions under which recovery will not be favorable:

1. Exacerbated symptoms triggered by topical ivermectin.
2. The patient's primary symptoms are papules, which typically take 3–9 months or an average of 4.5 months, to completely clear such symptoms.
3. In the event that papulopustules improve upon anti-*Demodex* treatment but are not completely removed, the following should be considered:
   (a) the anti-*Demodex* efficacy is insufficient,
   (b) the length of treatment is insufficient,
   (c) *Demodex* has developed drug resistance, and
   (d) rosacea is combined with other conditions causing facial pustules, such as eosinophilic pustular folliculitis (EPF), a peculiar scattered superficial pustular folliculitis which does not fit the symptoms of the well-known pustular dermatosis of the face, or acne vulgaris.

#### 3.3.8.1 *Exacerbation in the early stage of treatment*

The first issue which may be encountered is of exacerbation in the early stage of treatment, which was touched upon in the previous section when discussing how the accumulation of dead *Demodex* in hair follicles within the first week of treatment can trigger an immune response. In the first week, a weak steroid is applied to existing papulopustules or those that have developed through the treatment of topical ivermectin, which reduces the exacerbation rate from 12.8% to 1.4%; however, it is important to temporarily halt the treatment of topical ivermectin while continuing to use the topical steroid in the event of an increase in pustules, facial flushing, or new areas of erythema. The weakest or weaker steroid can continue to be applied locally to the exacerbated areas, and ivermectin treatment can be resumed once these areas have recovered. In this case, we recommend a half finger tip unit dosage to begin with, which should then be slowly increased to the size of one finger tip unit, after which point ivermectin treatment should be continued until papulopustules have been cleared completely. The immune response is typically aimed at *Demodex*, shown by the early exacerbation associated with ivermectin cream being typically followed by a sharp decline in DMD. With appropriate treatment, the clinical outcome will be positive.

#### 3.3.8.2 *Papules are difficult to treat*

Among individuals with PPR, there is a group whose disease manifests solely with papules. These patients have an unpredictable clinical outcome and a relatively high incidence of exacerbation in the early stages of treatment with ivermectin cream. We analyzed ten patients with papular rosacea, all of whom were women aged between 28 and 58 years, with a mean ± standard deviation of 44.4 ± 7.6 years of age. All of these patients exhibited a high DMD, and eight patients were associated with the treatment of topical ivermectin. Among these patients, two patients had large number of papules and erythema on both the fourth day and 17th day after treatment with ivermectin cream. Histopathological analysis revealed granulomatous dermatitis with an accumulation of epithelioid histiocytes and Langhans giant cells. The remaining six patients with papular rosacea experienced the exacerbation of their papules or erythema after treatment with ivermectin cream, with dosages ranging from half a finger tip unit to two finger tip units of cream. All six patients were administered with a weak topical steroid for the treatment of the papules in the first week. Among ten patients, we were unable to follow-up two patients, but among the remaining eight patients, six experienced complete or almost complete elimination of papules by the end of treatment, with a treatment duration of 2–8 months (average: 4.75 months). These six patients all were treated with doxycycline; another drug (indomethacin) was effective for one patient and ineffective for another patient; doxycycline combined with indomethacin was effective for two additional patients. Oral isotretinoin was used by only one patient who took 10–20 mg once per day for 15 weeks, but the results were not ideal. In summary, our preliminary recommendations for the treatment of papular rosacea are to first use doxycycline for 1 month to alleviate papules before the treatment of ivermectin cream, which should be introduced at a low dosage. Early application of low-dosage topical steroids is still useful in the treatment of papules (Figure 103).

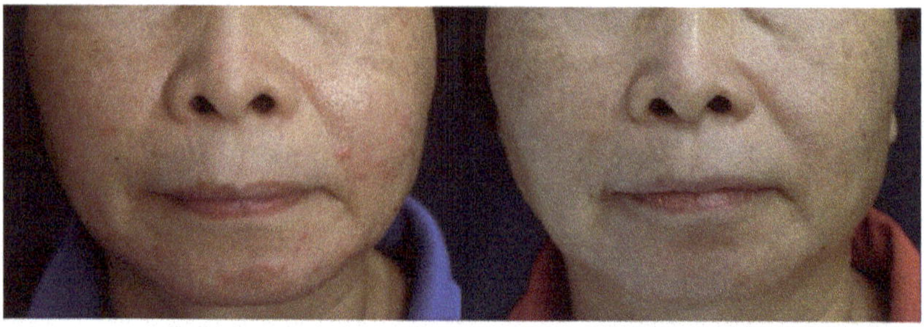

Pretreatment 2.5 months

**Figure 103.** A 56-year-old woman with fixed erythema and papules was administered with doxycycline, fexofenadine, ivermectin cream, and a weak steroid. After 6 weeks, her papules had disappeared, but her *Demodex* density was still as high as 128/cm$^2$. After administering 20-mg isotretinoin per day for 4 weeks, she was examined to have no *Demodex*.

### 3.3.8.3 *Unsatisfactory anti-Demodex effect and Demodex resistance*

First, when five pea-sized doses of topical ivermectin are used twice a day, *Demodex* can be reduced by 75% in 1 week, 67% in 2 weeks, 77% in 3 weeks, 78% in 4 weeks, and 85% in 5 weeks (Figure 101). When the number of *Demodex* mites is not reduced to at least 50% in a month, the rate of *Demodex* death is not as fast as expected. To increase the extermination effects, increasing the dosage of topical ivermectin should be considered. Second, combined treatment of topical ivermectin and oral carvedilol can increase the rate of *Demodex* death.[24] Third, the extension of the treatment duration can also increase its efficacy. Fourth, in some patients, isotretinoin can reduce the size of the *Demodex* within 2 weeks, with smaller *Demodex* mites being easier to exterminate. Finally, combined treatment of ivermectin and another anti-*Demodex* drug (such as permethrin) can increase the treatment efficacy in some of my cases.

### 3.3.8.4 *Rosacea combined with other facial pustular conditions*

Papulopustules are not exclusively the symptoms of rosacea. Other facial pustular conditions include EPF, bacterial folliculitis, superficial pustular folliculitis of the face, and acne vulgaris (Figure 104). Of these conditions, EPF is the most easily overlooked. Currently, none of the patients

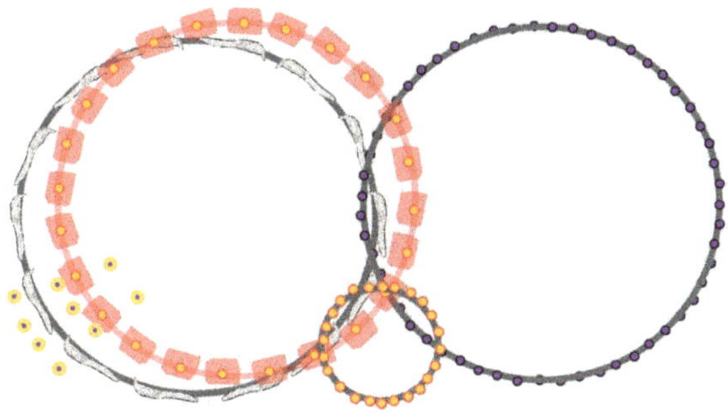

| | |
|---|---|
| | Papulopustular demodicosis |
| | Rosacea (erythema and papulopustules) |
| | Acne vulgaris |
| | Superficial pustular folliculitis of the face and neck |
| | Eosinophilic pustular folliculitis |

**Figure 104.** Papulopustular conditions of the face may occur concurrently or at different times; thus, an accurate differential diagnosis is necessary for treatment efficacy and preventing overtreatment.

with rosacea and EPF have experienced annular patches or postinflammatory hyperpigmentation typically associated with Ofuji's disease.[45] We have observed patients presenting with many discrete, tiny, superficial follicular pustules on the face that appear distinct from known facial dermatoses with pustules. We describe this condition as superficial pustular folliculitis of the face and neck.[44] Patients being treated for rosacea and *Demodex* should be considered for a biopsy or indomethacin treatment if they experience partial improvement but with more papules remaining than pustules.

### 3.3.9 *Is isotretinoin necessary for treating rosacea?*

Of my patients with rosacea and a high DMD, some patients were administered with isotretinoin. In an analysis of 80 patients, 14 patients were administered with isotretinoin; among the 14 patients, 5 patients took it at the beginning (including one patient with rhinophyma) and the other 9 patients took it in their late treatments. This is because five cases developed *Demodex* resistance, and the other four cases exhibited a rapid increase in *Demodex* over a short duration. Indeed, a precise treatment can be achieved, provided that *Demodex* is precisely assessed before and after treatment, with the TSM being highly recommended for such assessment.

### 3.3.10 *Advice for women with rosacea who are pregnant or preparing for pregnancy*

For women with rosacea who have been confirmed via microscopic testing to have a high DMD, safety during pregnancy or when preparing for pregnancy is crucial. Concerns exist regarding the safety of topical ivermectin for fetuses, and studies have shown that the transdermal absorption half-life can last as long as 6.5 days when such patients were administered with topical ivermectin once per day for 28 days. In our clinic, we have encountered patients who experienced a miscarriage because of the use of such medication. Pregnant women should use permethrin cream or metronidazole gel. Although the efficacy of these drugs is less ideal, they are Category B drugs and, therefore, relatively safe.

Women with rosacea who try for pregnancy should use permethrin or metronidazole gel. They may also consider birth control for a month while using 1-g topical ivermectin (the size of 2–2.5 finger tip units in women) in the morning and evening to have the opportunity to reduce *Demodex* until only 3% remain. Although high-dosage topical ivermectin has satisfactory therapeutic effect and short treatment period, preventive measures must be taken to avoid potential exacerbation of pustules.

## 3.4 Dr. Huang's process of diagnosing and treating rosacea

### 3.4.1 *Recommended process for diagnosis and treatment of facial papulopustules*

The author propose a flow chart of management of facial papulopustules (Figure 105). The diagnosis of rosacea is clear when a patient experiences papulopustules on the center of the face, centrofacial erythema which may

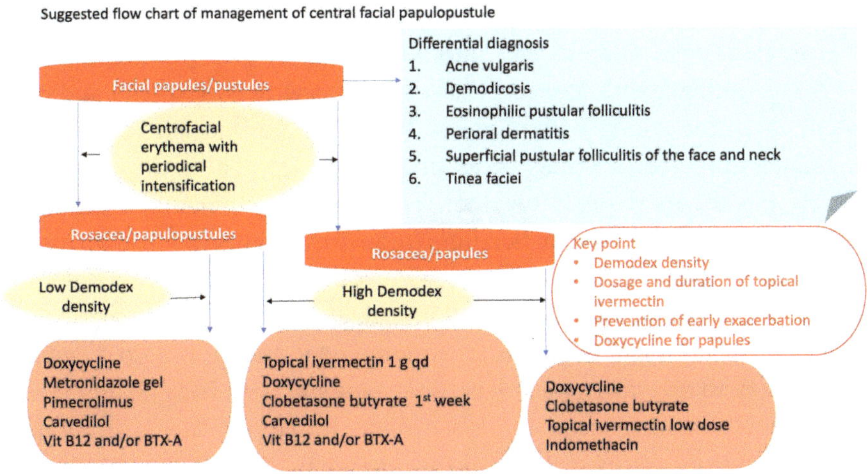


**Figure 105.** Recommended process for the diagnosis and treatment of facial papulopustules. In patients with both centrofacial papules and pustules and centrofacial persistent erythema which may be induced or periodically intensified by trigger factors, treatment should be considered based on *Demodex* density and papules/papulopustules separately. It is important to prevent the early exacerbation caused by anti-*Demodex* treatment. Management of erythema is not discussed here, as erythema and flushing in these patients are often less visible.

periodically intensified by trigger factors. There are several other papulopustular conditions that encroach the center of the face, but they lack the symptoms of the rosacea erythema. The conditions include acne vulgaris, characterized by whiteheaded and blackheaded comedones; demodicosis, which tends to lack the background erythema, facial flushing, and telangiectasia; EPF, also known as Ofuji's disease, is often marked by annular patches and postinflammatory hyperpigmentation, though we have also published reports regarding cases associated with demodicosis; perioral dermatitis, which is usually located around the mouth and nose areas; superficial pustular folliculitis of the face, which is an yet unclassified condition unrelated to *Demodex* that does not respond to acne vulgaris treatment; and tinea faciei. There are numerous diagnostic and treatment methods that cannot be covered here. In the event that a patient experiences papulopustular demodicosis and facial superficial pustular folliculitis with facial erythema, they should be followed up to check whether their condition changes into ETR.

Some patients with rosacea visit our clinic with widespread and persistent erythema, along with papules. These papules may be scattered or may cluster together and may be as small as the tip of a needle or may be densely packed as if fused together. This type of papular rosacea has a relatively high likelihood of leading to an increased growth of papules when treated with ivermectin cream, and even when exacerbation does not occur, the treatment duration may be extended for 3–6 months. For patients with papular rosacea, it is recommended to first use doxycycline for 1 month to alleviate papules before treatment with ivermectin cream, which should be introduced at a low dosage. Early application of low-potency topical steroids is still useful for treatment.

We can divide patients with PPR into two groups based on DMD. Patients with low DMD ($<12/cm^2$ examined by the TSM) should be administered with topical metronidazole or pimecrolimus based on phenotype to treat their papulopustules. Those with high DMD can be further divided into a papulopustular group and a purely papular group. For the former, topical ivermectin is recommended at a dosage the amount of two finger top units applied every evening and supplement with a low-potency steroid for early intervention in the first week to avoid progression of exacerbation. Carvedilol or doxycycline could also be added to reduce to the incidence of early exacerbation. Persistent erythema and facial flushing in these patients can be treated using hydroxocobalamin, intradermally injected BoNT-A, pulsed dye lasers, long-pulsed 532-nm laser, intense pulsed light, and microneedling bipolar pulsed radiofrequency. In the purely papular rosacea group, doxycycline should first be used for 1 month until the papules are alleviated, and then low-dose ivermectin cream should be used. The use of low-dose topical steroids in the first week can also be beneficial to reducing papules. Indomethacin can also be introduced to increase efficacy in case of coexistence of EPF.

If 80% of patients with papular rosacea experience exacerbated symptoms using ivermectin cream, why not remove the drug from their treatment plan to solve this problem? This is actually incorrect. Of our ten patients, one patient had chosen to avoid treatment with ivermectin cream for 1–2 years, and their condition had steadily deteriorated in that time.

Ultimately, we had to target *Demodex* to completely clear their papules. In conclusion, the key points for the treatment of PPR are as follows: (1) DMD must be assessed prior to treatment to decide on the direction of treatment. After treatment, it must be confirmed that DMD has dropped to standard levels before discontinuance of topical ivermectin to ensure a prolonged period during which symptoms are alleviated and treatment is not needed. (2) The dosage and treatment duration must be chosen appropriately in accordance with the circumstances and needs of each individual patient, and the treatment duration must be long enough to reduce *Demodex* to normal value. (3) To prevent early exacerbation of symptoms caused by ivermectin cream, a low-potency steroid can be prescribed as an early intervention for a flare, and doxycycline or carvedilol can be used simultaneously. (4) Patients with papular rosacea should be administered with doxycycline or oral isotretinoin.

### 3.4.2 *Key treatment details of rosacea erythema warranting special attention*

In addition to rosacea with centrofacial erythema, there are various differential diagnoses for central facial erythema. Fixed erythema with corresponding exacerbation trigger is a characteristic of rosacea (Figure 106) that can be tested using the arithmetic and isometric hand grip tests to induce flushing and assist with diagnosis (Figure 107). The global ROSCO panel recommends treatment based on phenotype (Table 11). Dr. Huang's approach is focused on the fact that there are triggers for rosacea, and even in rosacea with very obvious triggers. Some triggers may be preventable, whereas those that are not preventable include *Demodex*, thermal stimulation, and emotional stress. These factors can be treated by focusing on the target within the pathological pathway. In our patients with mild to moderate rosacea and a high DMD, the treatment is focused on decreasing DMD.

Approximately 64% of our patients were reduced to CEA grade 1 after treatment and did not require any further treatment. These patients also remained at grade 1 for a long time subsequently. For patients with hypertension, systolic blood pressure should be controlled to ≤120 mmHg, and the use of calcium channel blockers should be avoided, and clinically, amlodipine is

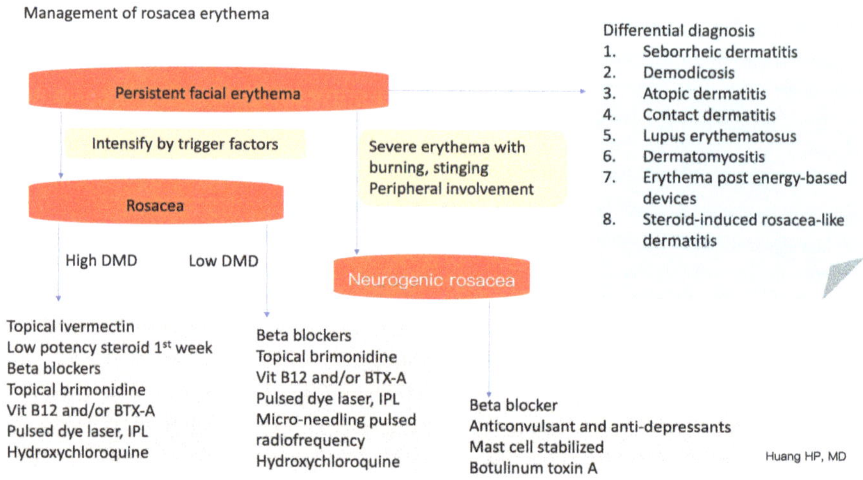


**Figure 106.** Differential diagnosis and treatment of rosacea erythema. Centrofacial persistent erythema, which may be intensified by trigger factors, enables the diagnosis of rosacea. In case with a high *Demodex* mite density (DMD) ivermectin cream may be added to the other treatments for erythema.

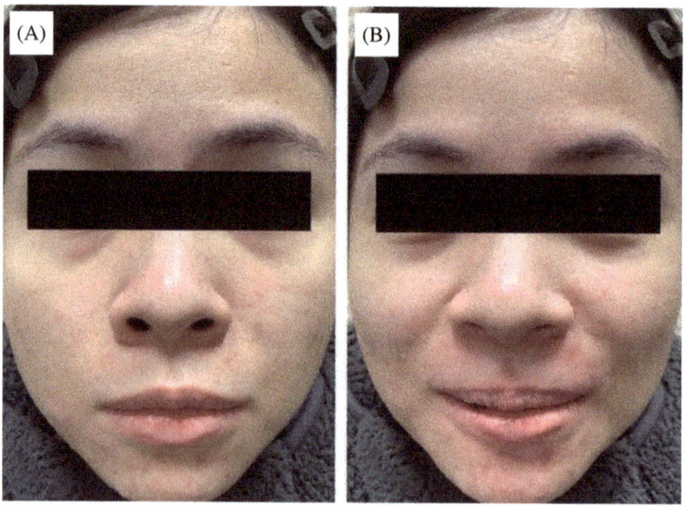


**Figure 107.** Facial flushing induced by the arithmetic test. (A) A patient with acne vulgaris who also presented with slight centrofacial erythema. (B) During a series of subtraction tests, the facial flushing clearly intensified, indicating that the patient also has rosacea.

most commonly used in Taiwan. Patients should avoid sources of heat, hot food, and hot drinks, but hydroxocobalamin can be used to inhibit prolonged flushing in patients who are unable to avoid thermal stimulation.

For patients willing to receive BoNT treatment, BoNT can block the skin sympathetic cholinergic response induced by exercise, whole body heating, and systemic thermal stimulation or stress and afferent sensory nerve response activated by local heat and cold stimuli which leads to facial flushing and can inhibit the release of mast cell granules.[46] Carvedilol and propranolol have good efficacy in patients facing stress and anxiety. A period of relative stability can be achieved using IPL, PDL, yellow lasers, and long-pulsed 532-nm laser. There are also new emerging treatments, such as bipolar microneedling radiofrequency, which have shown adequate efficacy.

Patients with rosea and prominent stinging or burning sensation are classified as those with neurogenic rosacea, which requires neurological or psychiatric treatment, and can be administered with anticonvulsants and antidepressants.[47] Approximately 84% of patients had a favorable response to these treatments.[48] Although the mechanism of stinging and burning in rosacea is not fully understood. The Aδ-fibers of sensory nerve are responsible for stinging pain, while C fibers carry burning sensation.[49] Axonal reflex triggered by topical capsaicin leads to antidromic release of substance P from C fiber and initiate burning sensation.[50] Substance P and calcitonin gene-related peptide (CGRP) excites nociceptors. Minute subcutaneous injection of substance P and CGRP elicits pain.[51] Substance P can activate mast cells leading to degranulation of tryptase, TNF, PGD2, and neurotrophins that may further activate C fiber.[52] Studies show that there are increased nerve densities and elevated levels of neurotransmitters, such as substance P, CGRP, PACAP, and VIP, in the dermis of rosacea skin (Figures 21–23). In patients with rosacea and prominent stinging and/or burning sensations, hyperexcitable or overactive Aδ and/or C fibers may theoretically be present. The triggering mediators of these fibers may be secreted from afferent sensory nerves, skin sympathetic cholinergic nerves, and mast cells. Mast cell degranulation is SNAP-23–dependent; SNAP-25 is primarily neuronal and, at most, shows weak/variable mRNA in some mast-cell preparations without convincing protein-level support.[53,54]

Treatments for neurogenic rosacea target signal transmission of Aδ and/or C fibers at the central nervous system level using gabapentinoids or through the inhibition of exocytosis with botulinum toxin A that cleaves SNAP 25 protein in the afferent sensory nerves, skin sympathetic cholinergic nerves, and thereafter indirectly suppresses mast cell activation by inhibiting the release of substance P.[55] These treatments are effective in alleviating stinging and burning sensations and erythema (Figure 108). In a series of 13 patients with neurogenic rosacea, complete or partial responses were observed with the aforementioned treatments (Table 18).

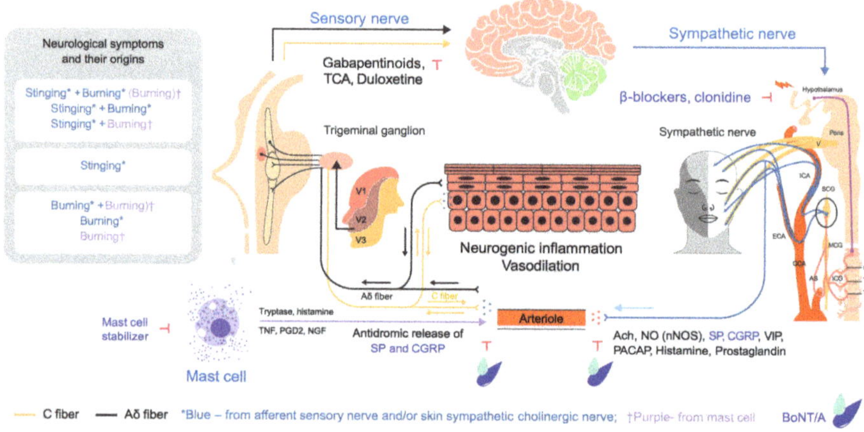


**Figure 108.** Theoretical pathogenesis of neurogenic rosacea. Activation of skin sympathetic cholinergic nerve via increase of core body temperature by stress or exercise leads to release of acetylcholine, nitric oxide, substance P, VIP, CGRP, PACAP, histamine and prostaglandins. Heat and cold stimuli activate afferent sensory nerve causing axonal reflex and antidromic release of substance P and CGRP. Substance P and LL-37 activate mast cell resulting in degranulation and release of tryptase, histamine, TNF, PGD2, and neurotrophins. Patients with neurogenic rosacea may have hyperexcitable or overactive Aδ and C fibers in the rosacea skin. Substance p from axonal reflex or skin sympathetic cholinergic nerve and mediators from mast cell may activate C fiber then initiate burning sensation. Substance P and CGRP excites nociceptors. Aδ fiber carries signal of stinging pain. Gabapentin, pregabalin, tricyclic antidepressants and duloxetine inhibit the stinging and burning sensation at the CNS level. At the skin level, botulinum toxin A blocks the transmission of axonal reflex and skin sympathetic and degranulation of mast cell by cleaving SNAP 25 protein. β-blockers and clonidine decrease the sympathetic activity. Mast cell stabilizers play an important role in relieving burning sensation from the mast cell origin. * indicates stinging and burning sensation from nerve origin. † indicates burning sensation from mast cells. Tinging and burning marked in blue indicate arising from nerves. Burning marked in purple indicates arising from mast cell.

**Table 18.** Summary of 13 patients with neurogenic rosacea

| No. | Phenotypes | Trearment | Sessions of BoNTA | Efficacy (Clearance of burning/stinging, CEA 0-1) | Timing of stinging or burn | Follow up (stable more than one year) |
|---|---|---|---|---|---|---|
| 1 | Burning, stinging, edema | Gabapentin, carvedilol, ketotifen, pine bark extract | No | Buring subsided, edema decreased | | Maintenance treatment |
| 2 | Burning, stinging | Doxycycline, propranolol, pregabalin, Vit B12, Dysport intradermal, Ketotifen | 2, (4 weeks apart) | Effective and reappeared after 3 weeks (life span of mast cells) | | Lost follow-up |
| 3 | Burning, stinging, itching | Dysport, pregabalin, duloxetine, carvedilol, Vit B12, estrogen | 2, (10 weeks apart) | Effective | All day long | Relieved for 1 year |
| 4 | Burning, stinging | Botox, carvedilol, pregabalin, Vit B12 | 1 | Effective | | Lost follow-up |
| 5 | Burning, stinging | Pregabalin, ketotifen, Dysport | 1 | Effective | For 10 years | Totally resolved |
| 6 | Stinging | Carvedilil, Soolantra, Vit B12, (Botox+ PDL)X3 | 3, (8 weeks apart) | Effective and lasted for 1 year | | Relieved for 1 year |
| 7 | Burning | Ketotifen, carvedilol | No | Burning subsided | Early morning | Lost follow-up |

*(Continued)*

**Table 18.** *(Continued)*

| No. | Phenotypes | Trearment | Sessions of BoNTA | Efficacy (Clearance of burning/stinging, CEA 0-1) | Timing of stinging or burn | Follow up (stable more than one year) |
|---|---|---|---|---|---|---|
| 8 | Burning | Botox (30,30,30,25,30U) Total 5 sessions every month | 5, (4 weeks apart) (Relapse of burning) | Effective and lasted more than 1 year | Bed time | Relieved for 1 year |
| 9 | Burning | Botox every 2 months for 10 sessions, pregabalin, clonidine | 10, (8 weeks apart) (Fear of relapse) | Effective (according to patient's request) | | Stable |
| 10 | Burning | Ketotifen, carvedilol, NO inducer, Dysport | 1 | Burning subsided | Day and bed time | Stable |
| 11 | Burning | Dysport | 3, (1 month and 3 months) | Effective | | Low grade relapse |
| 12 | Burning | Botox, carvedilol, sollantra, levocetirizine | 2, (10 months apart) | Burning subsided for 10–12 months | All day long | Stable |
| 13 | Burning | Pregabalin, Soolantra, Botox 25U, carvedilol, oral metronidazole, hydroxychloroquine, zolpidem | 1 | Burning subsided after Dysport | | Low grade relapse |

Patients with erythema who experience a burning and stinging sensation, or nocturnal flushing, are typically more difficult to treat and require an optimized treatment. Ketotifen, a mast cell stabilizer relieves nocturnal flushing in some of my cases. Hydroxychloroquine inhibits mast cell activation and infiltration, resulting in adequate treatment efficacy for those with ETR and PPR.

### 3.4.3 *Summary of rosacea diagnosis and treatment*

Differential diagnosis of rosacea may appear to be simple, but it is not. Various conditions and comorbidities must be identified and extracted to clarify the basis for treatment. Although the global ROSCO panel recommends treatment according to phenotype, we have found that identifying and eliminating the pathogenic cause, such as *Demodex*, and targeting treatment at the pathogenic pathways and targets associated with the cause typically lead to favorable treatment efficacy and a long duration during which the results of treatment are sustained. Although the results of anti-*Demodex* treatment are highly satisfactory in papules and pustules, the process is risky with an early flaring, which is preventable. Based on a retrospective statistical analysis of our clinical data, we have subdivided various conditions and recommended optimal principles of treatment to achieve the best possible results (Figure 109). Rosacea erythema and flushing act very similarly to the ebb and flow of the tides. The facial erythema we see with the naked eye is actually a sign of two neuronal and three non-neuronal vasodilation i.e., the sympathetic cholinergic vasodilation, afferent sensory vasodilation, prolonged vasodilation, immune-associated vasodilation and other non-neural vasodilation including vascular adhesion molecules (Figure 23). Treatment of this condition requires a multifaceted and complementary approach (Figure 110) and will be difficult to achieve if only a single treatment option is relied upon.

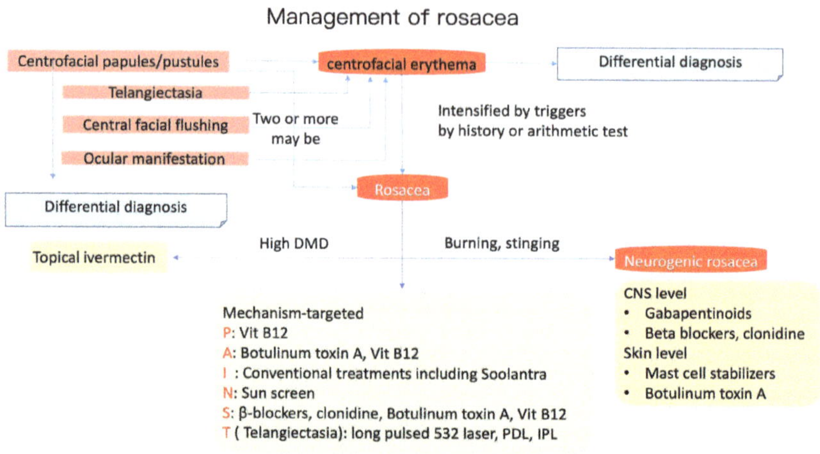


**Figure 109.** Management of rosacea. The first step is differential diagnosis, followed by the classification according to *Demodex* density, neurologic symptoms and phenotype. A multifaceted and mechanism-targeted treatment is suggested to stabilize rosacea. P indicates prolonged vasodilation. A indicates afferent sensory vasodilation and inflammation. I indictes immune-associated inflammation and vasodilation. N indicates other non-neural vasodilation and inflammation including vascular adhesion molecules. S indicates skin sympathetic cholinergic vasodilation and inflammation. Vit B12 prefers hydroxocobalamin. CNS, central nervous system. DMD, *Demodex* mite density. IPL, intense pulsed light. PDL, pulsed dye laser.

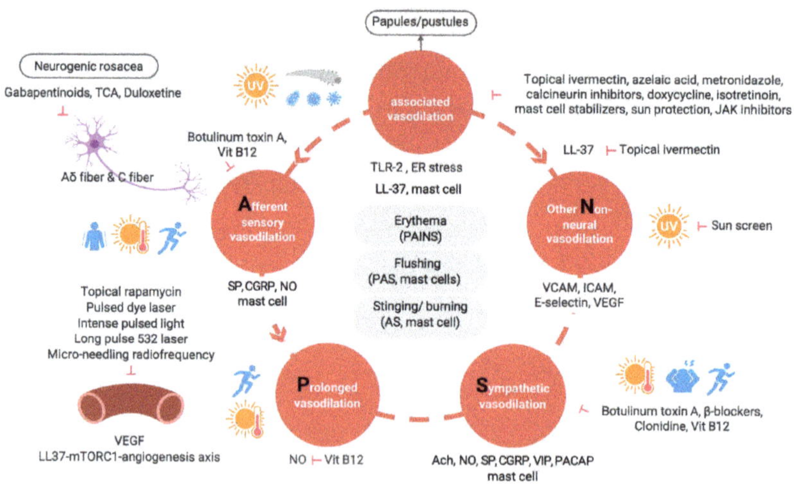


**Figure 110:** Pathway-level and targeted treatment for rosacea. Given the presence of five components of vasodilation and inflammation and telangiectasia, multiple targeted treatments are required stepwise or simultaneously for rosacea skin.

## References


1. Tan J, Almeida LM, Bewley A, et al. Updating the diagnosis, classification and assessment of rosacea: recommendations from the global ROSacea Consensus (ROSCO) panel. *Br J Dermatol.* 2017;176(2):431–438.
2. Schaller M, Almeida LMC, Bewley A, et al. Recommendations for rosacea diagnosis, classification and management: update from the global ROSacea COnsensus 2019 panel. *Br J Dermato*l. 2020;182(5):1269–1276.
3. van Zuuren EJ. Rosacea. *N Engl J Med.* 2017;377(18):1754–1764.
4. Miyachi Y, Imamura S, Niwa Y. Anti-oxidant action of metronidazole: a possible mechanism of action in rosacea. *Br J Dermatol.* 1986;114(2): 231–234.
5. Miyachi Y. Potential antioxidant mechanism of action for metronidazole: implications for rosacea management. *Adv Ther.* 2001;18(6):237–243.
6. Gollnick H, Layton A. Azelaic acid 15% gel in the treatment of rosacea. *Expert Opin Pharmacother.* 2008;9(15):2699–2706.
7. Crawford KM, Russ B, Bostrom. Pimecrolimus for treatment of acne rosacea. *Skin Med.* 2005;4(3):147–150.
8. Bamford JT, Elliott BA, Haller IV. Tacrolimus effect on rosacea. *J Am Acad Dermatol.* 2004;50(1):107–108.
9. Woo YR, Lim JH, Cho DH, Park HJ. Rosacea: molecular mechanisms and management of a chronic cutaneous inflammatory condition. *Int J Mol Sci.* 2016;17(9).
10. Kim JH, Oh YS, Choi EH. Oral azithromycin for treatment of intractable rosacea. *J Korean Med Sci.* 2011;26(5):694–696.
11. Dispenza MC, Wolpert EB, Gilliland KL, et al. Systemic isotretinoin therapy normalizes exaggerated TLR-2-mediated innate immune responses in acne patients. *J Invest Dermatol.* 2012;132(9):2198–2205.
12. Jackson JM, Knuckles M, Minni JP, Johnson SM, Belasco KT. The role of brimonidine tartrate gel in the treatment of rosacea. *Clin Cosmet Investig Dermatol.* 2015;8:529–538.
13. Logger JGM, Olydam JI, Driessen RJB. Use of beta-blockers for rosacea-associated facial erythema and flushing: a systematic review and update on proposed mode of action. *J Am Acad Dermatol.* 2020;83(4):1088–1097.
14. Wu AK, Liu FF, Xie HF, et al. Clinical features and risk factors for nasal rosacea: a hospital- based retrospective study. *Dermatol Ther.* 2021;11(6): 1953–1963.

15. Chang DK, Savetsky IL, Avashia YJ, Rohrich RJ. A safe, modern treatment of rhinophyma: the 5-step technique. *Plast Reconstr Surg Glob Open.* 2020;8(6):e2620.
16. Oliveira CMM, Almeida LMC, Bonamigo RR, Lima CWG, Bagatin E. Consensus on the therapeutic management of rosacea — Brazilian Society of Dermatology. *An Bras Dermatol.* 2020;95(Suppl 1):53–69.
17. Hampton PJ, Berth-Jones J, Duarte Williamson CE, et al. British Association of Dermatologists guidelines for the management of people with rosacea 2021. *Br J Dermatol.* 2021;185(4):725–735.
18. Salleras M, Alegre M, Alonso-Usero V, et al. Spanish consensus document on the treatment algorithm for rosacea. *Actas Dermosifiliogr.* 2019;110(7):533–545.
19. Kellogg DL, Jr., Pérgola PE, Piest KL, et al. Cutaneous active vasodilation in humans is mediated by cholinergic nerve cotransmission. *Circ Res.* 1995;77(6):1222–1228.
20. Kellogg DL, Jr. In vivo mechanisms of cutaneous vasodilation and vasoconstriction in humans during thermoregulatory challenges. *J Appl Physiol.* 2006;100(5):1709–1718.
21. Huang YW, Huang HP, Hsu CK, Lee JY. Hydroxocobalamin: an effective treatment for flushing and persistent erythema in rosacea. *J Clin Aesthet Dermatol.* 2022;15(6):42–45.
22. Metzler-Wilson K, Toma K, Sammons DL, et al. Augmented supraorbital skin sympathetic nerve activity responses to symptom trigger events in rosacea patients. *J Neurophysiol.* 2015;114(3):1530–1537.
23. Schaller M, Gonser L, Belge K, et al. Dual anti- inflammatory and antiparasitic action of topical ivermectin 1% in papulopustular rosacea. *J Eur Acad Dermatol Venereol.* 2017;31(11):1907–1911.
24. Huang HP, Hsu CK, Lee JY. Rosacea with persistent facial erythema and high *Demodex* density effectively treated with topical ivermectin alone or combined with oral carvedilol. *Dermatol Ther.* 2021;34(2):e14899.
25. Koçak M, Yali S, Vahapolu G, Ekiolu M. Permethrin 5% cream versus metronidazole 0.75% gel for the treatment of papulopustular rosacea. A randomized double-blind placebo-controlled study. *Dermatology.* 2002;205(3):265–270.
26. Atif M, Estrada-Mondragon A, Nguyen B, Lynch JW, Keramidas A. Effects of glutamate and ivermectin on single glutamate-gated chloride channels of the parasitic nematode H. contortus. *PLoS Pathog.* 2017;13(10):e1006663.

27. Huang HP, Hsu CK, Lee JY. Topical ivermectin-induced transient flare of rosacea as a host reaction to killed *Demodex* mites preventable by short-term use of topical corticosteroid. *Dermatol Ther.* 2022;35(7):e15517.
28. Zhang J, Jiang P, Sheng L, et al. A novel mechanism of carvedilol efficacy for rosacea treatment: toll-like receptor 2 inhibition in macrophages. *Front Immunol.* 2021;12:609615.
29. de Ménonville ST, Rosignoli C, Soares E, et al. Topical treatment of rosacea with ivermectin inhibits gene expression of cathelicidin innate immune mediators, LL-37 and KLK5, in reconstructed and ex vivo skin models. *Dermatol Ther.* 2017;7(2):213–225.
30. Zhang X, Song Y, Ci X, et al. Ivermectin inhibits LPS-induced production of inflammatory cytokines and improves LPS-induced survival in mice. *Inflamm Res.* 2008;57(11):524–529.
31. Wong BJ, Hollowed CG. Current concepts of active vasodilation in human skin. *Temperature.* 2017;4(1):41–59.
32. Herborn KA, Graves JL, Jerem P, et al. Skin temperature reveals the intensity of acute stress. *Physiol Behav.* 2015;152(Pt A):225–230.
33. Alawi KM, Aubdool AA, Liang L, et al. The sympathetic nervous system is controlled by transient receptor potential vanilloid 1 in the regulation of body temperature. Faseb J. 2015;29(10):4285–4298.
34. Moura AKA, Guedes F, Rivitti-Machado MC, Sotto MN. Inate immunity in rosacea. Langerhans cells, plasmacytoid dentritic cells, Toll-like receptors and inducible oxide nitric synthase (iNOS) expression in skin specimens: case-control study. *Arch Dermatol Res.* 2018;310(2):139–146.
35. Rochelle LG, Morana SJ, Kruszyna H, Russell MA, Wilcox DE, Smith R. Interactions between hydroxocobalamin and nitric oxide (NO): evidence for a redox reaction between NO and reduced cobalamin and reversible NO binding to oxidized cobalamin. *J Pharmacol Exp Ther.* 1995;275(1):48–52.
36. Coleman JW. Nitric oxide: a regulator of mast cell activation and mast cell-mediated inflammation. *Clin Exp Immunol.* 2002;129:4–10.
37. Li Y, Xie H, Deng Z, et al. Tranexamic acid a meliorates rosacea symptoms through regulating immune response and angiogenesis. *Int Immunopharmacol.* 2019;67:326–334.
38. Bageorgou F, Vasalou V, Tzanetakou V, Kontochristopoulos G. The new therapeutic choice of tranexamic acid solution in treatment of erythematotel-angiectatic rosacea. *J Cosmet Dermatol.* 2019;18(2):563–567.

39. Zhong S, Sun N, Liu H, Niu Y, Chen C, Wu Y. Topical tranexamic acid improves the permeability barrier in rosacea. *Dermatol Sin.* 2015;33(2): 112–117.
40. Kim SJ, Park JY, Shibata T, Fujiwara R, Kang HY. Efficacy and possible mechanisms of topical tranexamic acid in melasma. *Clin Exp Dermatol.* 2016;41(5):480–485.
41. Taieb A, Khemis A, Ruzicka T, et al. Maintenance of remission following successful treatment of papulopustular rosacea with ivermectin 1% cream vs. metronidazole 0.75% cream: 36-week extension of the ATTRACT randomized study. *J Eur Acad Dermatol Venereol.* 2016;30(5):829–836.
42. Huang HP, Hsu CK, Lee JY. Thumbnail-squeezing method: an effective method for assessing *Demodex* density in rosacea. *J Eur Acad Dermatol Venereol.* 2020;34(7):e343–e345.
43. Taieb A, Ortonne JP, Ruzicka T, et al. Superiority of ivermectin 1% cream over metronidazole 0.75% cream in treating inflammatory lesions of rosacea: a randomized, investigator-blinded trial. *Br J Dermatol.* 2015; 172(4):1103–1110.
44. Huang HP, Huang CM, Hsu C-K, Yang C-C, Lee J. Superficial Pustular Folliculitis of the Face and Neck — A Non-Infectious Eruption Responding to Topical Steroids. *J EADV clinical practice*. 2025;4:1057–1067.
45. Huang HP, Hsu CK, Chao SC, Yang CC, Chen GS, Lin CH, Huang CM, Lee JY. Eosinophilic pustular folliculitis associated with *Demodex* overgrowth or demodicosis on the face – A report of five cases. *Dermatol Sin.* 2021;39: 132–136.
46. Choi JE, Werbel T, Wang Z, Wu CC, Yaksh TL, Di Nardo A. Botulinum toxin blocks mast cells and prevents rosacea like inflammation. *J Dermatol Sci.* 2019;93(1):58–64.
47. Scharschmidt TC, Yost JM, Truong SV, Steinhoff M, Wang KC, Berger TG. Neurogenic rosacea: a distinct clinical subtype requiring a modified approach to treatment. *Arch Dermatol.* 2011;147:123–126.
48. Kim HO, Kang SY, Kim KE, Cho SY, Kim KH, Kim IH. Neurogenic rosacea in Korea. *J Dermatol.* 2021;48:49–55.
49. Yam MF, Loh YC, Tan CS, Khadijah Adam S, Abdul Manan N, Basir R. General Pathways of Pain Sensation and the Major Neurotransmitters Involved in Pain Regulation. *Int J Mol Sci.* 2018;19.

50. Cotton P. Studying selective blockage of sensation. *JAMA*. 1990;264:14–15.
51. Dafny N. Pain Principles. https://nba.uth.tmc.edu/neuroscience/m/s2/chapter06.html
52. Stassen M, Hartmann AK, Delgado SJ, Dehmel S, Braun A. Mast cells within cellular networks. *J Allergy Clin Immunol*. 2019;144(4S):S46–S54.
53. Woska JR, Jr., Gillespie ME. SNARE complex-mediated degranulation in mast cells. *J cell Mol Med*. 2012;16:649–656
54. Sander LE, Frank SP, Bolat S, Blank U, Galli T, Bigalke H, et al. Vesicle associated membrane protein (VAMP)-7 and VAMP-8, but not VAMP-2 or VAMP-3, are required for activation-induced degranulation of mature human mast cells. *Eur J Immunol*. 2008;38:855–863.
55. Wang L, Wang YJ, Hao D, Wen X, Du D, He G, et al. The Theranostics Role of Mast Cells in the Pathophysiology of Rosacea. *Front Med (Lausanne)*. 2019;6:324.

# 4

# Skin Care

## 4.1 Skin care for patients with rosacea

Rosacea can be improved through basic skin care, avoiding exacerbating factors, and treatment.

Patients with rosacea present a substantial challenge to dermatologists because of their sensitive skin, the need to control *Demodex* and the bacterial colonies, the instability of their vascular tone, the need for creams to conceal vasodilation, and the need to prescribe some treatments. Continuous and gentle skincare and effective use of cosmetics can lead to drastic improvements in rosacea. When choosing skincare products, patients should follow the primary principle of avoiding products which cause stinging, burning, or skin irritation. In a survey of 1,066 patients conducted by the NRS of the US, 41% reported that skincare products aggravated their condition and 27% stated that certain cosmetics caused their rosacea to flare-up.

Basic skin care can maintain the stability of skin, particularly cleansing, moisturizing, and sun protection. Products that are simple, with no pigments or fragrance should be used, and new products should be tested by applying a tiny amount on the peripheral skin of the face before applying to the entire face (such as on the neck or behind the ears). If the skin reacts, the ingredients should be noted and products with similar ingredients should be avoided as much as possible. Patients should also avoid frequently changing the products that they use on the face. Ingredients which commonly cause irritation should be avoided, including alcohol, witch hazel, camphor, fragrance, glycolic acid, lactic acid, menthol, eucalyptus oil, sodium lauryl sulfate, and urea. Creams should be chosen over lotions or gels, and toner and astringent creams should not be used. Patients with rosacea may have dry, normal, oily, or combination skin. Oily skin refers to oiliness across the entire facial skin, without patches of dryness. Dry skin refers to dry and tight skin, in some cases with areas of flaking skin, and with no patches of oiliness. Combination skin refers to a condition where the T-zone is quite oily and other areas of the face are normal or dry.

Proper moisturizer should be used according to the patient's skin condition. The ideal cleanser should leave the skin feeling clean but not dry. Those with normal skin should use a moisturizing lotion, whereas those with oily skin, such as patients with rosacea and seborrheic dermatitis or sebaceous hyperplasia, should choose a serum. Those with dry skin should use a cream-type product, and those with combined skin-types should treat different areas of their skin accordingly. Exfoliating products may damage the epidermal barrier and thus are unsuitable.

**Specific skincare products and cosmetics**

Because patients with rosacea have relatively sensitive skin, they should use skincare or cosmetic products with caution. For those with unstable rosacea, cosmetics should be avoided, but their use may be resumed upon the stabilization of the skin's condition. We recommend the use of dry powder products (pressed and loose powder) and avoid the use of ingredients with high oil content or relatively complex ingredients, such as liquid foundation, BB/CC/DD creams, toning cream, concealer, cushion foundations, primer, cleansing oils, and hair conditioner. Patients can use a green-tinted concealer combined with a skin tone concealer to cover facial flushing. It is also very important to ensure all cosmetics are properly cleaned after use.

### 4.1.1 *Skin cleansing*

Gentle cleansing can remove excess oils, environmental pollutants, bacteria, and other microorganisms, as well as the remnants of cosmetics or other skincare products. In recent years, studies have shown that excessive cleansing of the skin may lead to rosacea. A study of 3,439 college freshmen in China found a positive association between showering for more than 11 minutes (11 minutes, OR 2.60) and cleansing the face more than twice per day (≥2 times/day, aOR 1.70) with the development of rosacea.[1]

The NRS of the US has a range of detailed information regarding cleansing, moisturizing, sun protection, and cosmetics, which is worth consulting (https://www.rosacea.org/patients/skin-care-and-cosmetics). Choice of facial cleanser depends upon patient skin type. For dry to normal or combination skin, we recommend the use of a soap-free cleanser. For extremely dry skin, a creamy, nonfoaming, and soap-free cleanser is recommended. For oily skin, we recommend a gentle soap cleanser, avoiding any scrubbing motions, as vigorous rubbing or excessive cleansing can irritate the skin. Cleansing must always be done gently, using the fingertips and avoiding abrasive washcloths or sponges which may cause irritation. Because hot or cold water can cause facial flushing or irritation, the face should be rinsed with warm water. After cleansing, the face should be gently dried using a paper or cotton face towel. Topical medications should be applied after the face has dried completely. After applying medication, the patients should wait for 5–10 minutes before applying moisturizer, sunscreen, or cosmetic products.

### 4.1.2 *Moisturizer*

Moisturizer is key to preventing burning, prickling, itching, or irritation of the skin for individuals with rosacea and helps to build the epidermal barrier. Rosacea is often characterized by a diminished facial epidermal barrier, along with relatively high transepidermal moisture loss, both of which may make skin susceptible to sensitivity and inflammation.

Winter or dry weather can exacerbate the damage to already sensitive skin in patients with rosacea. The more severe a patient's inflammatory papulopustules, the greater is the need for moisturizer. Facial moisturizers have now been developed by experts to specifically aid patients with rosacea and are designed to calm and soothe the skin and aid in the prevention of redness caused by irritation. Some moisturizers even contain green coloring to help improve the appearance of facial flushing.

### 4.1.3 *Sunscreen*

In a survey by the NRS, 81% of patients believed that sun exposure was the primary trigger for their rosacea to flare. There are two types of UV rays: UVA, which causes the skin to age, and UVB, which causes sunburn. The use of mineral sunscreens which contain zinc oxide or titanium dioxide, with UVA/UVB protection of SPF 30 or above, are recommended and can help minimize irritation. Sunscreen should be applied every day, year-round, whether it is a sunny or overcast day. Some sunscreens are developed specifically for skin that is prone to redness, and may be tinted green or skin colored. This allows for protection from the sun's rays while helping reduce visible redness and can also act as a foundation. Individuals should apply sunscreen 30 minutes prior to going out into the sun to allow the skin time to absorb the product, and reapply once every 2 h if swimming or engaging in activities causing perspiration. In ideal circumstances, the individuals should avoid sun exposure, particularly during 10:00 h to 16:00 h when the sunlight is strongest. High altitude, snow, water, and even glasses can increase the effects of UV rays.

### 4.1.4 *Makeup*

Makeup can help instantly improve the external appearance of skin and increase self-confidence about one's own appearance. Prior to makeup, individuals should use skincare products suited to their skin type and should cleanse and moisturize the face. The higher the number of ingredients and products that are applied to the skin, the higher the likelihood of skin being burdened by such products. We recommend the use of multi-functional products to prevent such a burden. Green-tinted foundations containing SPF can be used to correct visible redness and even out skin tone. Oil-free foundations and concealers are easier to remove from the skin. The foundations should align with the natural skin tone as much as possible, while the concealers should be just one shade lighter than the natural skin tone.

### 4.1.5 *A message to men with rosacea*

We recommend that male patients with rosacea use electric razors for shaving to avoid irritation caused by dull blades, and any shaving creams or lotions causing burning or stinging sensation should be avoided. After shaving, such patients should use an aftershave moisturizer to help soothe the skin.

## 4.2 Avoiding trigger factors

Avoiding triggers is the key to maintain stable rosacea condition. The NRS previously conducted a questionnaire survey on the triggers of rosacea and found the top two triggers to be sun exposure (81%) and emotional stress (79%), which caused exacerbated symptoms in 80% of patients. Other triggers include weather (cold, hot, wind, and humidity), food (alcohol, hot drinks, and spicy food), and specific skincare products and cosmetics (see Section 1.3.4). Triggers will be different for each patient with rosacea; thus, it is not necessary to contraindicate every trigger detailed in this book. Instead, we recommend that individuals identify their personal rosacea symptom triggers and then selectively avoid such triggers. The key concept is focusing on targeting the bigger issues rather than the smaller ones, i.e., first deducing which triggers have a higher probability of exacerbating symptoms, and if symptoms remain exacerbated after eliminating those triggers, foods and other triggers with a relatively low probability should be recorded and avoided to ensure the lowest possible impact on quality of life.

### 4.2.1 *Avoiding sun exposure*

Although patients with rosacea should do their utmost to avoid triggers, this does not mean that they should completely stop doing things that they love. It is well known that sunlight can affect rosacea; thus, it is important to protect skin from sun exposure when such patients exercise outdoors. To protect oneself from the sun, we recommend the use of products such as hats, umbrellas, masks, sunscreen clothing, SPF 30+ sunscreen, and PA+++ sunscreen (UVA and UVB). However, some patients with rosacea may find that their skin is irritated by sunscreen. Therefore, we recommend that such patients prioritize the use of mineral sunscreens (zinc oxide and titanium dioxide). Mineral sunscreens can achieve the sunscreen effect through reflection, scattering, and refraction, whereas chemical sunscreen absorbs sunlight and converts it into heat, which can cause facial redness, flushing, and heat sensitivity in patients with rosacea. Moreover, chemical sunscreens may have a chemical composition that irritates the skin. During outdoor activities, we recommend the reapplication of sunscreen every 2 h. Waterproof or sweat-resistant sunscreens should be not used because such sunscreens can be very difficult to remove from the skin.

### 4.2.2 *Mood changes*

Emotional factors include stress and anxiety. We recommend patients to maintain a normal schedule of work and rest, avoid staying up too late, ease emotions, remove sources of anxiety, and regularly participate in interesting or relaxing activities; when experiencing mood changes, patients should immediately take deep breaths to help alleviate stress. Some patients take regular mirror photos or selfies to check the redness of their face, which may intensify stress. We recommend those patients avoid excessive focus on their face.

Anxiety triggers the “fight or flight response,” which involves the release of adrenaline into the bloodstream causing vasodilation. Anxiety causing issues with circulation can only be resolved by controlling the anxiety. Such patients can seek help from a psychiatrist or engage in indoor exercises, yoga, and massages to help improve their anxiety levels. Stress-induced erythema and flushing can be improved via the intradermal injection of BoNT. The pretreatment arithmetic and isometric grip strength tests are useful in screening for patients who would benefit from BoNT treatment.

### 4.2.3 *Weather*

When the weather is excessively hot, cold, or windy, rosacea symptoms can be triggered. Rosacea shares many similarities to a rose growing in a greenhouse, requiring specific care. The patients should remain in a cool and air-conditioned environment when the weather is too hot, keep warm when the weather is too cold, and avoid strong winds and dress in layers of clothing when the temperature is changing drastically. Indoor high-temperature environments such as saunas, hot showers, and steam baths should be avoided. For those who wish to enjoy time in a sauna, hot shower, or steam bath, vitamin B12 can be used to increase heat resistance.

### 4.2.4 *Exercise*

Symptoms of rosacea are often exacerbated by exercise, but this does not mean that those with rosacea must stop exercising, as exercise has both physical and psychological benefits. Patients with rosacea should find a form of exercise which suits their own condition and needs. Patients should consider avoiding high-intensity exercise or replacing a single long exercise session with multiple intermittent sessions. Some doctors recommend that patients walk briskly as opposed to running, as running often leads to redness of the cheeks. For patients with rosacea, swimming is a good choice of exercise because swimming does not result in excessive heat. It is still important to wash one's face and use moisturizer after swimming, as chlorinated water is alkaline, which can disrupt the naturally mild acidic pH of the skin, breaking the skin's barrier and leading to a feeling of tightness, dryness, and sensitivity. Low intensity exercises such as yoga and aqua aerobics are also good activities, which are beneficial for health.

The environment in which exercise is performed is also important. This should be in a cool environment such as a room with air conditioning, close to an electric fan, or outdoors in the early morning or evening when the weather is cooler. A cool and damp towel can be placed around the neck, or an atomizer bottle filled with cold water can be used to lower body temperature. Those with rosacea attempting to balance both physical health and facial health can choose BoNT and vitamin B12 treatment to increase their heat resistance during exercise (Figure 104).

For those yearning for unrestricted exercise, dual treatment of excessive redness and excessive heat is the solution. The primary mechanisms involved in the exacerbation of erythema in patients with rosacea include temporary flushing induced by cutaneous sympathetic activity, temporary flushing caused by the sensory nerves responding to thermal stimulation, and prolonged breakouts of flushing induced by NO. Depending on the intensity of the exercise, different degrees of treatment can be planned. The primary treatment consists of Dr. Huang's heat resistance treatment for rosacea.

### 4.2.5 *Food*

Patients should identify foods that exacerbate rosacea, which typically means avoiding hot foods, hot drinks, spicy flavors, and alcohol. Some patients may find their symptoms exacerbated by foods rich in histamin, (citrus fruits, pickles, nuts, and chocolate) or cinnamaldehyde (cinnamon, tomatoes, citrus fruits, and chocolate). Other triggering foods may include ginger, garlic, mustard, fried foods, animal livers, yogurt, cheese, soy sauce, yeast, and vinegar. We recommend that patients keep a food diary to identify foods that exacerbate rosacea symptoms and to maintain the results of rosacea treatment through proper dietary control. Because food contraindications have an incidence rate <13%, it is not necessary to prohibit the intake of all foods mentioned in this book. Instead, we recommend that individuals identify their personal rosacea symptom triggers and then selectively avoid such triggers.

### 4.2.6 *Rosacea diary*

Patients should consider maintaining a diary for recording daily weather, routine, exercise, and diet to identify under which conditions symptoms flare. This can help in identifying and avoiding potential triggers.

## 4.3 Treatment

Treatment can be broadly categorized into topical medications, systemic treatments, injectable medications, surgery, and photoelectric lasers. Choice of treatment should be primarily based on whether there is an excess of *Demodex*, the erythema exacerbation pathway, and the rosacea phenotype to ensure appropriate treatment. This has been discussed in detail in the previous chapter. The goal of treatment is to enable patients to return to a normal life similar to that of a healthy individual. To achieve such results from treatment, it is necessary to perform testing and evaluation prior to treatment to identify the triggering pathway and predict and test treatment efficacy. After treatment, it is important to evaluate opportunities for improvement and whether an additional dose or a prolonged treatment period is required.

## References

1. Zuo Z, Wang B, Shen M, et al. Skincare habits and rosacea in 3,439 Chinese adolescents: a university-based cross-sectional study. *Acta Derm Venereol.* 2020;100(6):adv0008
2. Plewig G, Melnik B, Chen W. Plewig and Kligman's acne and rosacea. Switzerland: Springer International Publishing; 2019. https://www.rosacea.org/

# 5

# About Ocular *Demodex* Infestation

## 5.1 Introduction to the disease

### 5.1.1 *Introduction*

In addition to infecting the skin, *Demodex* infestations can commonly infect the eye, leading to a number of diseases of the ocular surface. However, ocular *Demodex* infestation is often easily ignored and overlooked by patients themselves and even by ophthalmologists conducting diagnosis and treatment. It is a chronic inflammatory disease of the ocular surface and is highly correlated with anterior and posterior blepharitis, blepharoconjuncitvitis, and blepharokeratitis and may even affect anterior segment conditions. Severe *Demodex* infestations may even result in loss of sight. However, the impact of *Demodex* infestations on the eye, the role played by *Demodex* in ocular surface diseases, and the pathogenic mechanism all remain unclear. In addition, ocular *Demodex* infestations are still underdiagnosed and undertreated. Ocular *Demodex* infestations are directly proportional to age, with older age having an increased incidence of *Demodex*.

Ocular *Demodex* infestation may occur indirectly through hands or skin coming in contact with the bed sheets, blankets, or towels of someone with *Demodex*, or it may occur through *Demodex* spreading from the face of a person with pre-existing *Demodex* to the eyes of another individual. There are two main types of ocular *Demodex*. The first being *D. folliculorum*, which is around 0.4 mm in size and is found in the follicles of eyelashes and reaches imago-stage 1–2 weeks after hatching. This type of *Demodex* typically activates during the night, feeding on human skin cells. This causes follicular swelling and inflammation, or blepharitis, triggering epithelial hyperplasia, keratinization, and white dandruff-like flakes on the eyelashes. Meanwhile, this causes inflammation of the hair follicles primarily on the face and at the eyelash root and triggers epithelial hyperplasia and keratinization, resulting in the accumulation of cylindrical dandruff on the eyelashes. The second being *D. brevis*, which primarily lives within the meibomian gland on the rims of the eyelid inside the tarsal plate. *Demodex brevis* are around 0.3 mm in size and live in glands close to the hair follicles. They feed on the cells of eyelid glands, and in case of overgrowth, they block the opening to the sebaceous glands, resulting in abnormal oil secretion, which affects the oily layer of the tear film and causes dry eye syndrome (DES).

The two species of *Demodex* can be more accurately distinguished by the shape of their tails, with a blunt, fingertip-like tail being associated with *D. folliculorum*, and a sharp, cone-shaped tail being associated with *D. brevis* (See Section 1.3.3). Currently, the role played by ocular *Demodex* in the diseases of the eye surface is not fully clear. However, we do know that these *Demodex* often live in the sebaceous and meibomian glands, resulting in meibomian gland blockage, which in turn leads to decreased oil secretion. This leads to the excess evaporation of tears and may even lead to DES caused by insufficient oil. Blepharitis is typically associated with the blockage of oil in the meibomian glands and the occurrence of bacteria and inflammation. It can also be associated with improper cleaning of the eyelid (makeup and contact lenses), *Demodex*

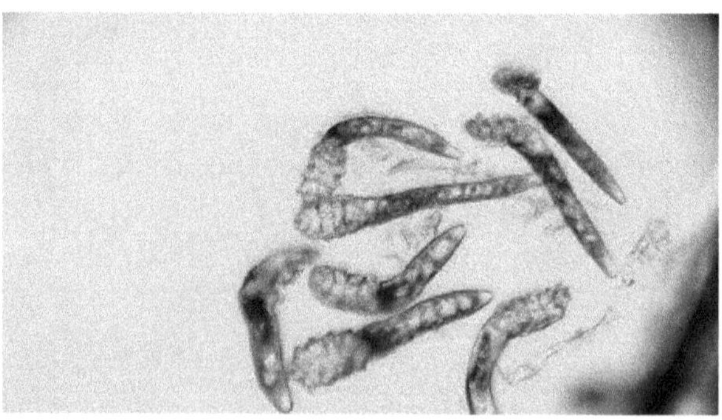

**Figure 111.** Microscopic view of *D. folliculorum* at the root of the eyelashes.

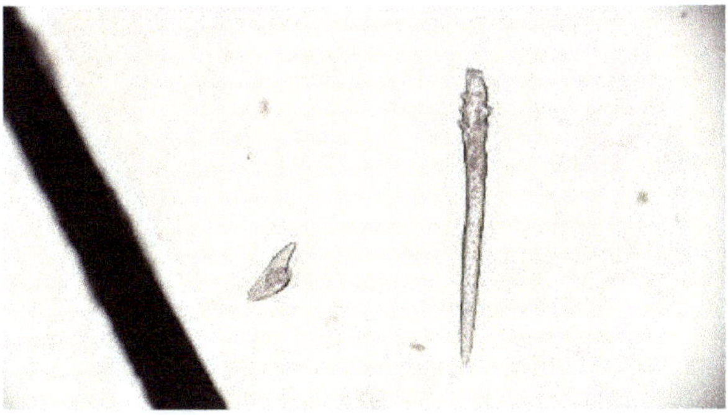

**Figure 112.** Microscopic view of *D. folliculorum* ovum and protonymph at the root of the eyelashes.

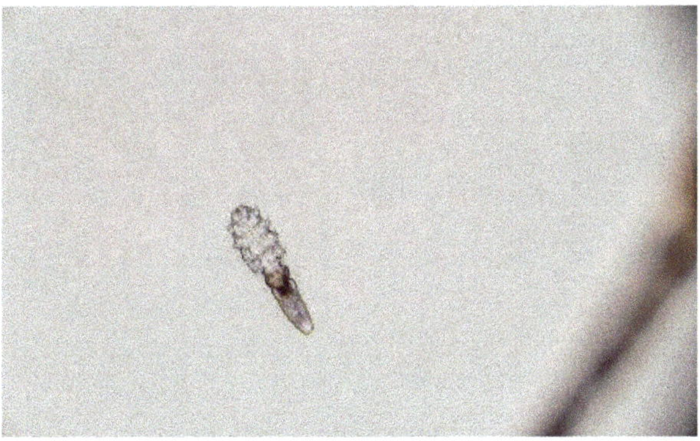

**Figure 113.** Microscopic view of *D. brevis* at the root of the eyelashes.

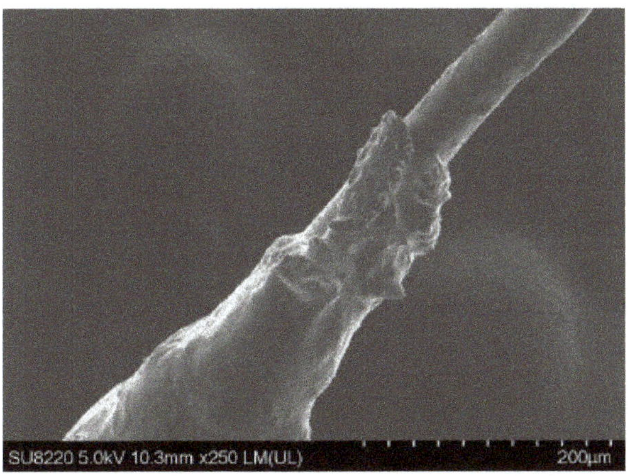


**Figure 114.** Clinical condition of ocular demodicosis observed via scanning electron microscope (SEM).

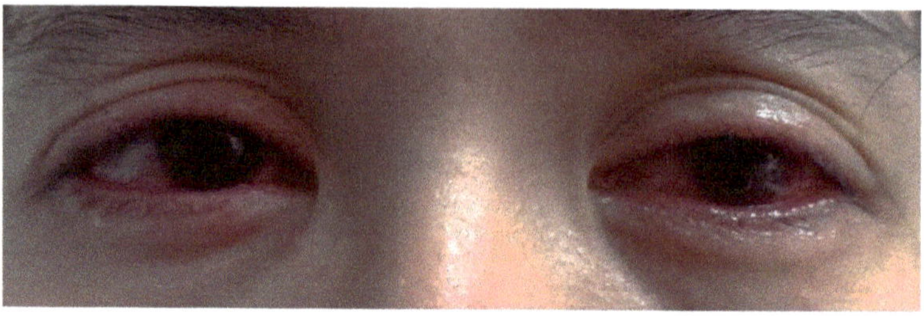

**Figure 115.** Clinical symptoms of ocular *Demodex* infestation.

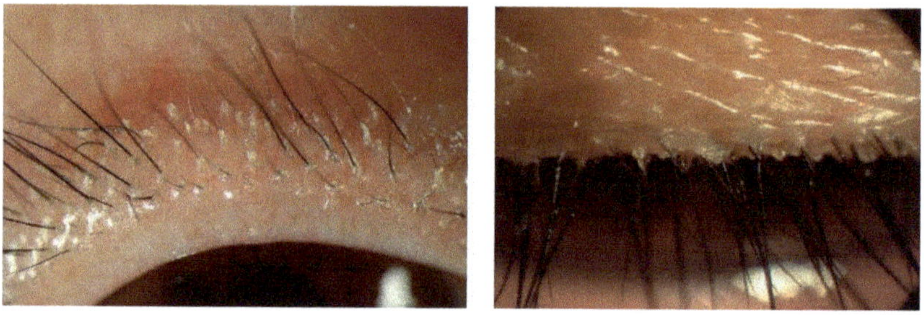

**Figure 116:** (1) *Demodex* blepharitis and (2) cylindrical dandruff (CD) accumulation.

infestations, seborrheic dermatitis, and chemical irritation (cosmetics or skincare products).

Ocular *Demodex* infestation mainly includes common clinical symptoms such as itching, burning, dryness, irritation, watering, foreign body sensation, crusting, lid margin redness, and blurry vision. However, as these symptoms are all nonspecific, they may be easily overlooked or classified as different ocular disorders.

Ocular *Demodex* infestation mainly includes common clinical signs such as cylindrical dandruff (CD), eyelash disorders, lid margin inflammation, meibomian gland dysfunction, blepharoconjunctivitis, and blepharokeratitis.

Even on eyelids that appear normal, a slit lamp may reveal the presence of *Demodex* eggs.

Although people are becoming increasingly aware of the dangers of *Demodex* to the eye, the biggest difficulty still lies in how to effectively and consistently eradicate *Demodex*, which even ophthalmologists commonly overlook.

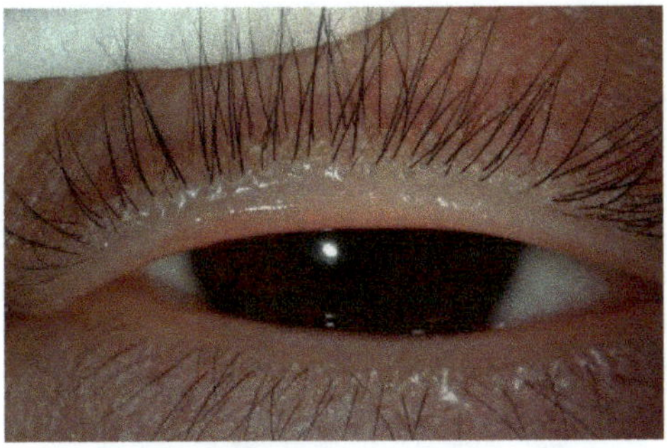

**Figure 117.** *Demodex* blepharitis and CD accumulation.

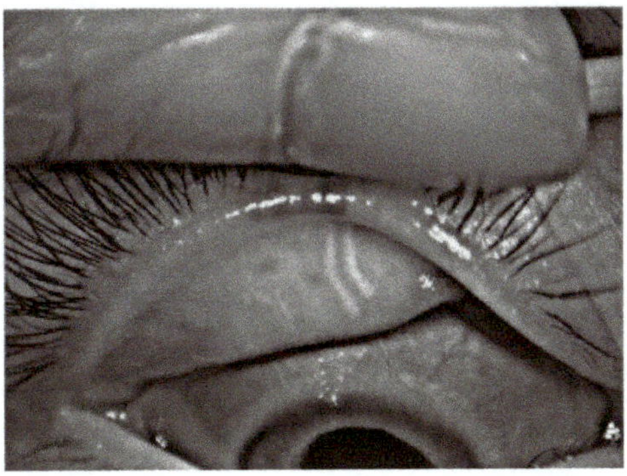

**Figure 118.** *Demodex* may cause obstruction of the meibomian glands, which can be detected using the OCULUS Keratograph® 5M to perform meibography.

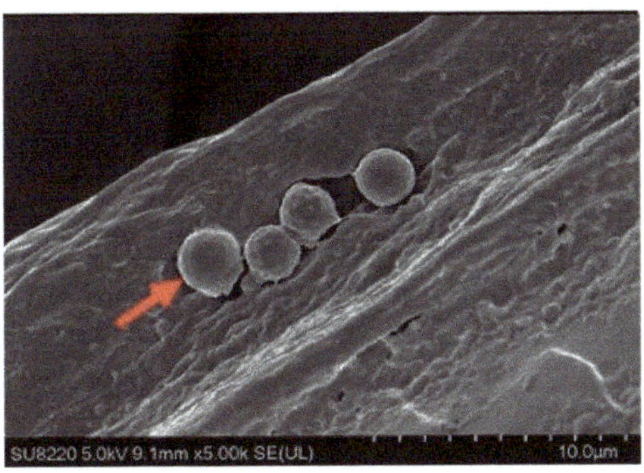


**Figure 119.** SEM image of *Demodex* eggs which may be found at the eyelash root.

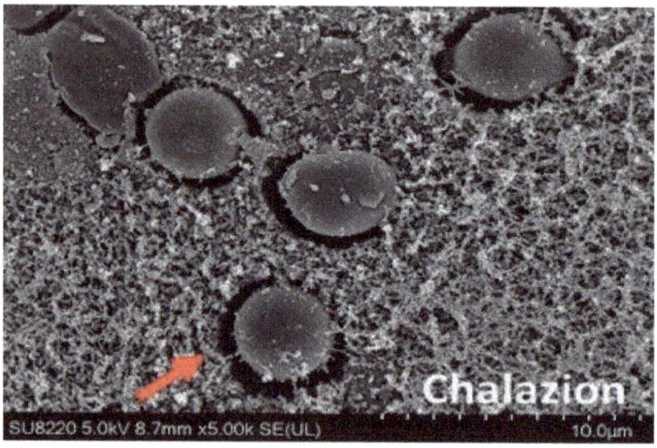


**Figure 120.** *Demodex* eggs may be found in the chalazion. Granulation tissue may be surgically removed. SEM image.

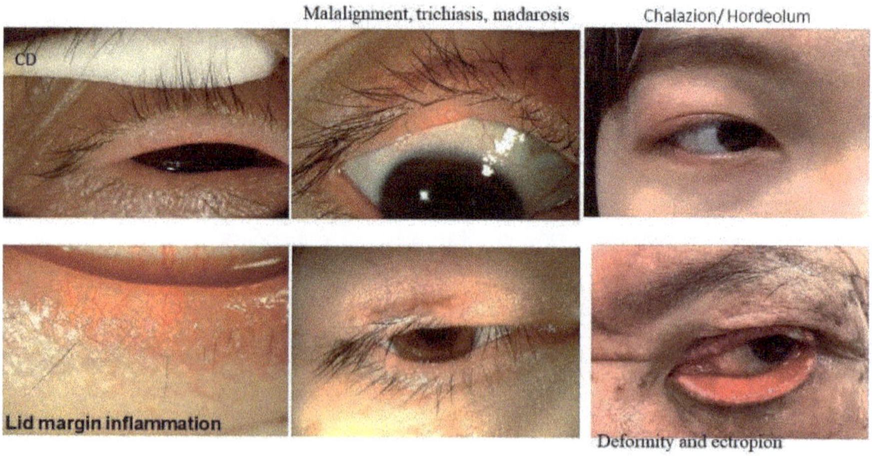


**Figure 121.** *Demodex* infestation of the eyelid causes eyelash disorders, including dandruff and secretions, lid margin inflammation, trichiasis, eyelid misalignment which leads to ectropion or entropion of the eyelid, meibomian gland dysfunction (MGD), hordeolum or chalazion, blepharoconjunctivitis, and blepharokeratitis.

Adult *Demodex* mate and lay eggs at the eyelash root or around the meibomian glands. However, the life cycle of *Demodex* lasts only a few weeks, with larvae taking 3–4 days to hatch and reaching maturity in around 7 days, meaning the life cycle lasts only around 14 days.[1]

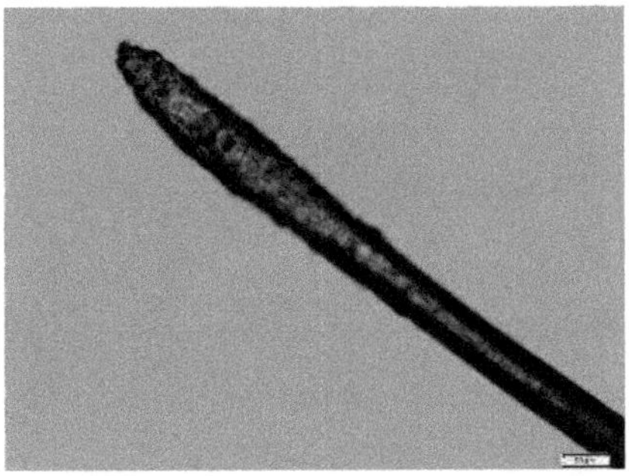

**Figure 122.** A healthy eyelash root without *Demodex* infestation.

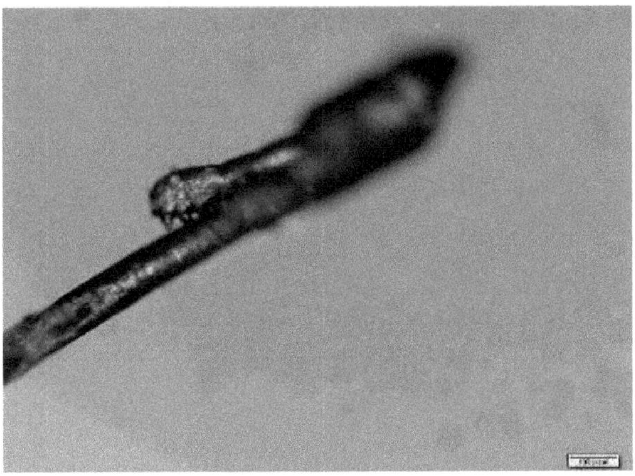

**Figure 123.** An eyelash root presenting the early stages of *Demodex* infestation.

## 5.2 Diagnosis of ocular *Demodex* infestations

### 5.2.1 *Differential diagnosis of ocular Demodex infestations*

Ocular *Demodex* infestations have key clinical signs, and diagnosis is often made based on the clinical signs, as opposed to clinical symptoms.

## 5.3 Treatment for ocular *Demodex* infestation

*Demodex folliculorum* is highly resilient to the external environmental factors and is well-adapted to a wide range of acidic and alkaline conditions.

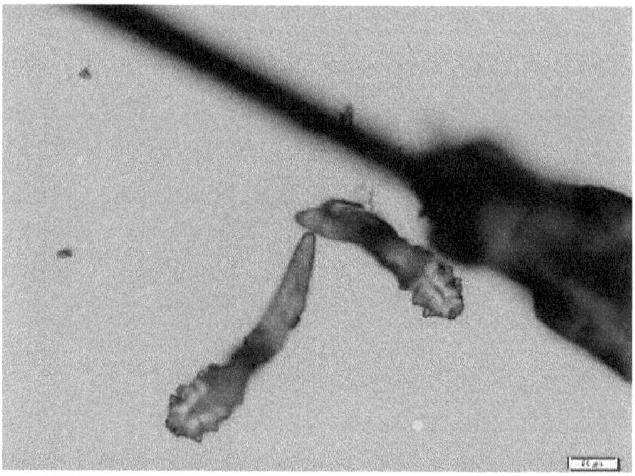

**Figure 124.** *Demodex* at the eyelash root.

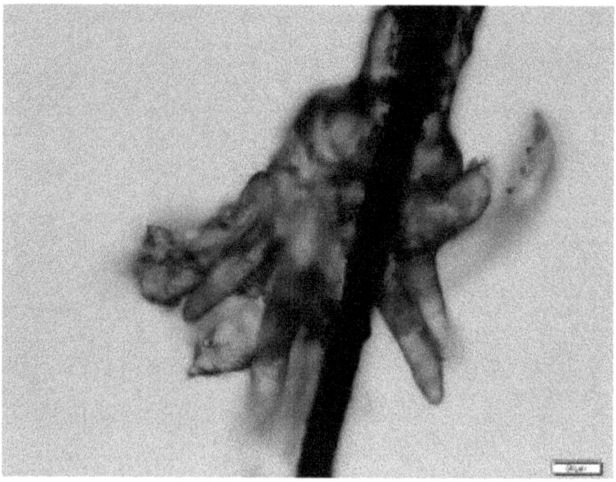

**Figure 125.** Numerous *Demodex* individuals breeding at the eyelash root.

The types of soap and baby shampoo used daily cannot kill these mites. Cleaning: The active ingredient of tea tree oil terpinen-4-ol can effectively kill *Demodex* and remove dandruff, secretions, and waste matter from *Demodex*. *Demodex* are averse to the scent of tea tree oil; thus, it can help move them out of the hair follicles. Hot compress: *Demodex* are incredibly sensitive to temperature changes, with temperatures <0 °C and >37 °C being

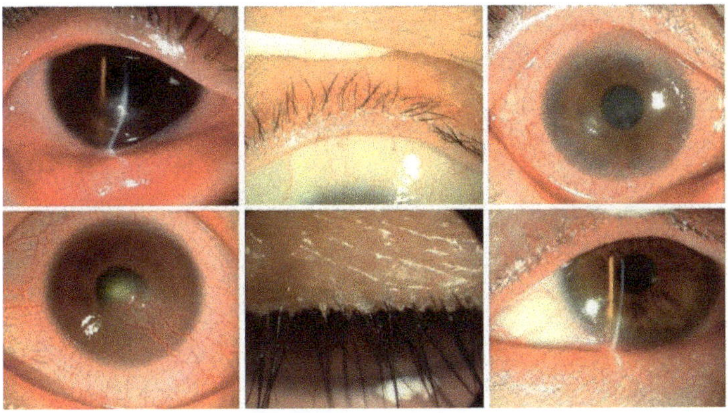

**Figure 126.** Common clinical signs of ocular *Demodex* infestation.

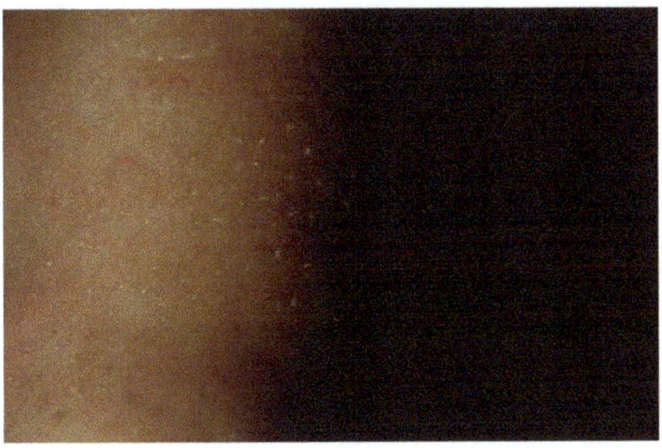

**Figure 127.** Clinical signs of facial demodicosis.

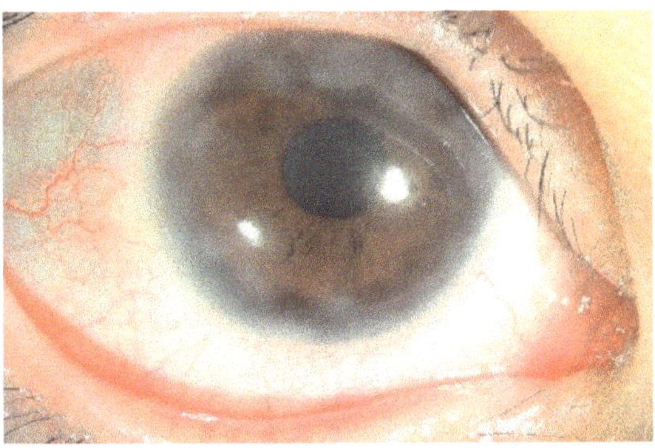

**Figure 128.** Damage to the corneal periphery caused by *Demodex* infestation.

unsuitable for survival, 54 °C capable of killing *Demodex*, and 58 °C capable of effectively eliminating the mites. A hot compress between 40 °C–50 °C can be used as a supplementary treatment for *Demodex*.

**Cleaning:**

**Eyelid cleaning method**

1. Wash both hands, and avoid wearing contact lenses.
2. Use a sterilized cleansing cotton pad or cleansing mousse designed specifically for the eye (Figure 129).
3. Close both eyes gently to avoid wiping at the cornea (pupil of the eye) and gently lift the eyelid to reveal the root of the eyelash (eyelid) (Figure 130).
4. Move in a single direction from the inner to the outer corner of the eye and gently wipe along the eyelash root, ensuring to avoid a back-and-forth motion (Figure 130).
5. With eyes still closed, gently wipe around the perimeter of the eye.
6. Repeat the above procedure to clean the other eye. Do not use the same cotton pad for both eyes.

Reference (3–19)

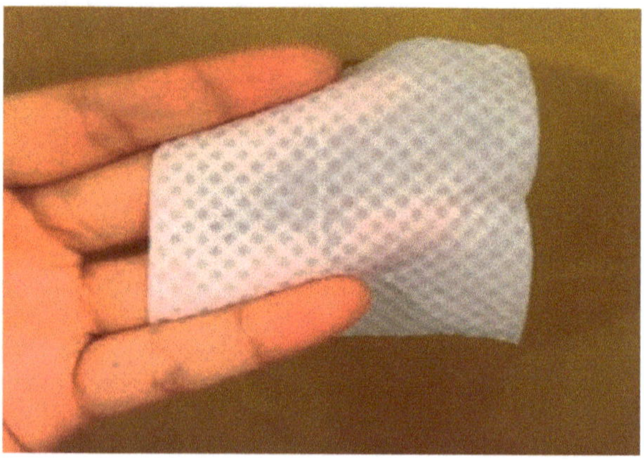

**Figure 129.** Cleansing pads.

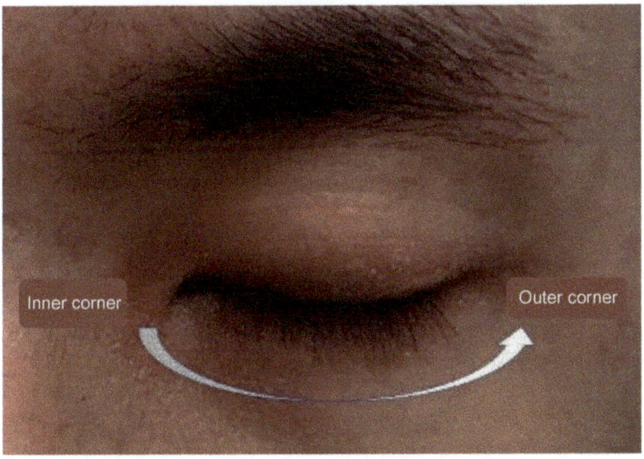


**Figure 130.** Wipe in a single direction.

**Hot compress:**

The benefits of the hot compress application are as follows:

1. Unblocking the meibomian glands, allowing tears to secrete as normal, and maintaining the stability of the lipid layer of the tear film.
2. Increasing blood circulation around the eyes, which improves metabolism.
3. Relieving fatigue and soreness of the eyes.
4. Relaxing the eye muscles and increasing visual accommodation.

A hotter hot compress than the normal does not indicate better efficacy. The ideal temperature range of a hot compress is 42 °C–45 °C for 10–15 minutes. According to the literature, maintaining the temperature of a hot compress at 45 °C for 4 minutes makes the effective temperature of the inner eyelid reach 40 °C. Maintaining the compress at 45 °C for 5 minutes every day for >2 weeks showed that it helped relieve DES, reduce eye fatigue,[4] and improve meibomian gland dysfunction (MGD).[5] Far infrared (FIR) and warming functions can promote blood circulation around the eye socket and relax the ciliary muscles, which helps eliminate eye fatigue and pain caused by swelling.[6,7] Of the many ways of applying a hot compress, patients can choose a safe, timed, and temperature controlled hot compress eye mask with medical device license. Patients may also use a clean towel that has been soaked in hot boiling water, though not hot enough to scald the hands, and wrung out. The wet towel is placed over the eyelids, while ensuring that the temperature is not too high and the towel is properly sterile to avoid eye infections. It is also important to avoid pressing against the eyeballs during the hot compress. We recommend the use of a hot compress twice per day for 10 minutes at a time.

**Tips for choosing a hot compress eye mask:**

1. Select hot compress eye masks with a medical device license approved by the Ministry of Health and Welfare.
2. Select hot compress eye masks which allow for a set temperature (up to 45 °C) and a set period (up to 10–15 minutes).
3. Select hot compress eye masks that have CE electrical safety qualifications and have undergone electromagnetic testing.
4. Select hot compress eye masks with FIR radiation functions.
5. Select reusable and rewashable masks.

**During the hot compress, the following should be noted:**

1. Remove contact lenses and clean off all makeup prior to the application of the hot compress.
2. If there are any prescribed medications or ointments which must be applied at a set time, use the hot compress before medication.
3. Regularly wash the hot compress eye mask to avoid secretions from the eye remaining on the mask and causing inflammation or bacterial infection.
4. Avoid excessively high temperature of the hot compress on the eyes, and maintain the temperature within the range of 40 °C–50 °C.
5. Avoid excessive pressure while wiping on the ocular area.
6. After the hot compress, use a specialized eyelid cleanser to remove discharges and dirt from the ocular area.
7. Ensure that the use of the hot compress eye mask is continued regularly.

**Drug treatment:**
Clinical experience has shown that although some patients may have no visible signs of blepharitis or *Demodex*, clinical indications and

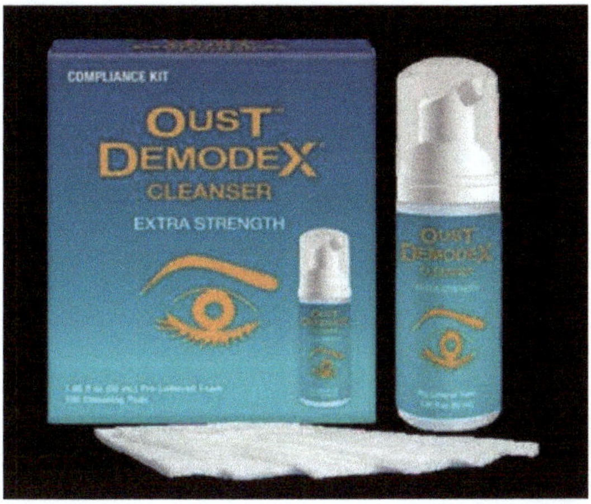


**Figure 131.** Cleansing cotton pads or cleanser for the eye area (containing tea tree oil).

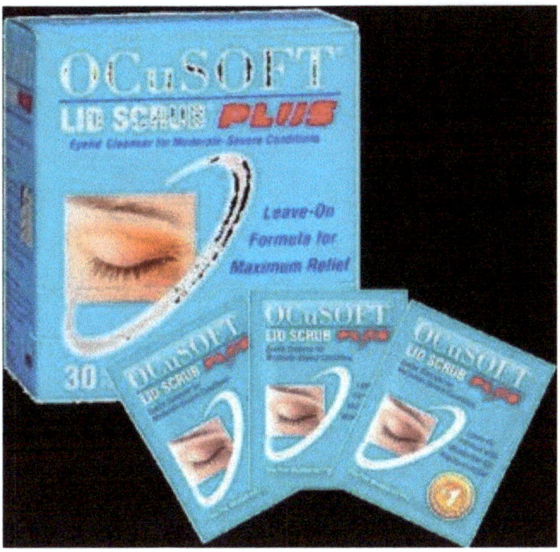


**Figure 132.** Cleansing cotton pads for the eye area (single-use packaging).

microscopic testing of plucked eyelashes show that *Demodex* is often found deep within the hair follicle; thus, it would be incorrect to rule out *Demodex*. Such varied manifestations of *Demodex* are because of each individual's facial cleansing habits. In terms of the strategy for the

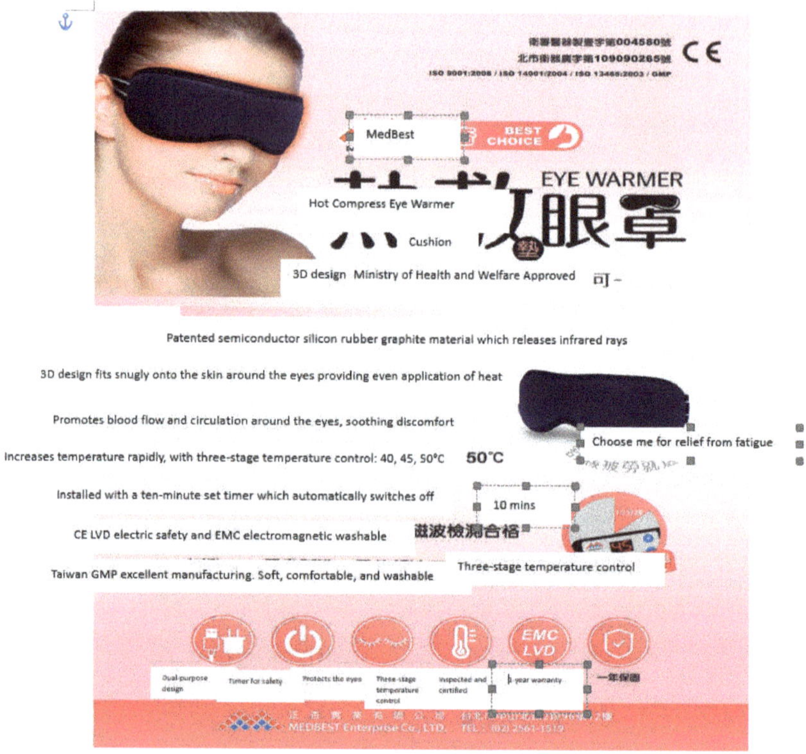


**Figure 133.** Hot compress eye mask.

treatment of *Demodex* infestations, the most important factor is to screen *Demodex* mites to identify patients with a *Demodex* infestation, find a method of halting the vicious cycle, and alleviate the clinical symptoms for the patients. However, because *Demodex* can hide deep into pores and eyelash follicles, medication is usually only able to eliminate *Demodex* closer to the surface. Relying solely upon medication for elimination will result in limited effectiveness; thus, we recommend that medication is combined with cleansing and hot compresses to bring *Demodex* to the surface where they can be killed. In addition to actively treating the condition with the help of an ophthalmologist, we recommend at-home eyelid cleansing to improve symptoms alongside treatment. This involves using dedicated cleansing products for the eye area and wiping them gently from the inner to the outer corner of the eye along the eyelash roots (see Figures) to remove secretions and oils from the eyelid and eyelash roots. *Demodex folliculorum* is highly resilient to the environmental factors. Traditional textbooks on the matter recommend the use of daily use products such as baby shampoo and soap, but such products are not effective at killing *Demodex*.[12] As shown in the literature, effective products for eliminating *Demodex* include tea tree oil[12–14] and octanediol.[14–18]

The active ingredient of tea tree oil, Terpinen-4-ol, can effectively kill *Demodex* at a concentration >1% (12) and can remove dandruff, secretions, and waste matter from *Demodex*. *Demodex* are averse to the scent of tea tree oil, so it can help move them out of the hair follicles. However, tea tree oil can be irritating to the eyes, and therefore is unsuitable for patients to administer it directly. After consultation with a specialized

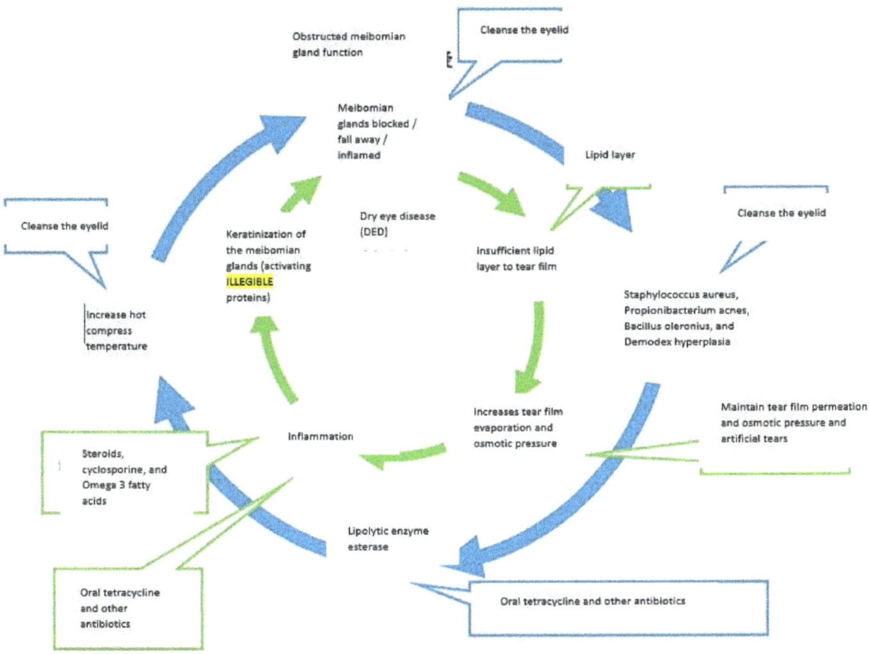


**Figure 134.** The treatment strategy is based upon the principle of first confirming and diagnosing the existence of *Demodex* infestation, then treating the underlying diseases such as DES or MGD, breaking the vicious cycle of *Demodex*, and keeping the ocular surface in good condition.

References: *Br J Ophthalmol*. 2016; 100: 300–306.[3]

ophthalmologist, individuals are recommended to buy ophthalmologist-approved diluted tea tree essential oil prepared as an eyelid cleansing solution. The eyes should be cleansed once each morning and evening for at least 4 weeks to reduce *Demodex* infestation numbers.[14]

On a daily basis, in addition to cleansing the eyelids, hygiene habits should also be improved. Towels, bedsheets, and pillowcases that are used on a daily basis should be regularly cleaned and changed. Such habits can be combined with the use of a hot compress at 40 °C–50 °C for 10–15 minutes. This range of temperature is not conducive to *Demodex* survival. Therefore, the method is a supplementary to treating *Demodex* infestations (19).

# 6

# About Ocular Rosacea

## 6.1 Introduction to the disease

### 6.1.1 *Introduction*

Ocular rosacea is an inflammation of the ocular surface causing redness, burning, or itching. Ocular rosacea is often found concomitant with facial rosacea or other chronic facial skin conditions. Sometimes, ocular rosacea is the first symptom to appear before the progression to facial rosacea. Ocular rosacea typically occurs in adults from 30 to 50 years of age. Ocular rosacea is typically found in patients with existing skin conditions such as rosacea, but it is also possible to experience ocular rosacea alone. Facial rosacea has a higher incidence of affecting women than men, whereas ocular rosacea is more likely to affect men than women.

Although the causes of ocular rosacea are unclear, it can be associated with heredity, environmental factors, bacterial involvement, obstructed eyelid glands (such as meibomian glands), ocular Demodex infestations, and, according to some scholars, *Helicobacter pylori* infection, the primary bacterium causing gastric and duodenal ulcers. There are also some factors that aggravate facial rosacea, which also aggravates the condition of ocular rosacea. Possible risk factors are as follows: hot or spicy food or drink, alcohol, sunlight, wind, extreme temperature, stress, anger, embarrassment, other strong emotions, intense exercise, hot baths, and saunas.

## 6.2 Symptoms

### 6.2.1 *Symptoms of ocular rosacea (Subtype 4)*

The clinical signs and symptoms of ocular rosacea (subtype 4) may precede, coincide with, or follow the occurrence of facial rosacea symptoms, or ocular symptoms may also occur in isolation. The severity of ocular rosacea symptoms may differ from facial rosacea severity.

Another important factor in the diagnosis of ocular rosacea is whether ocular Demodex infestations also occur. Such infestations are relatively common but are easily overlooked by ophthalmologists during differential diagnosis. The primary symptom of ocular Demodex infestation is redness, heat, itchiness, dryness, foreign body sensation, and other common nonspecific symptoms seen in ophthalmology. More severe symptoms than the aforementioned symptoms may also occur, such as dandruff, inflammation, and chronic ulcers. In some cases, patients may even experience corneal perforation leading to the release of aqueous humor, vision loss, and even blindness. As the symptoms of this condition are typically nonspecific, the majority of patients are underdiagnosed and undertreated. To identify the affected patients, the first step involves assessing the patient for blepharitis, checking the roots of the eyelashes for Demodex, and looking for typical signs such as the existence of CD. However, the

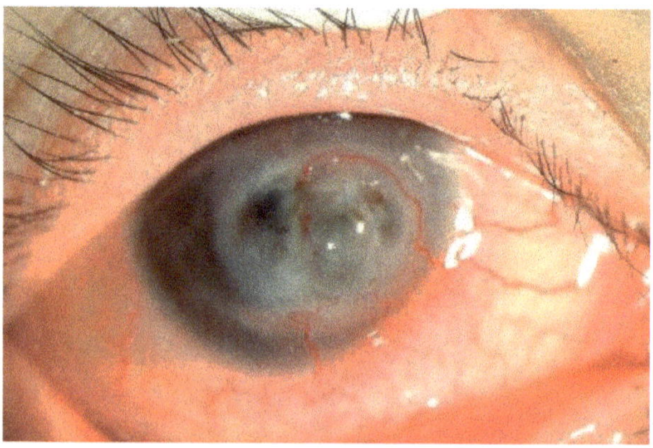

**Figure 135.** Ocular rosacea can damage the ocular surface tissues.

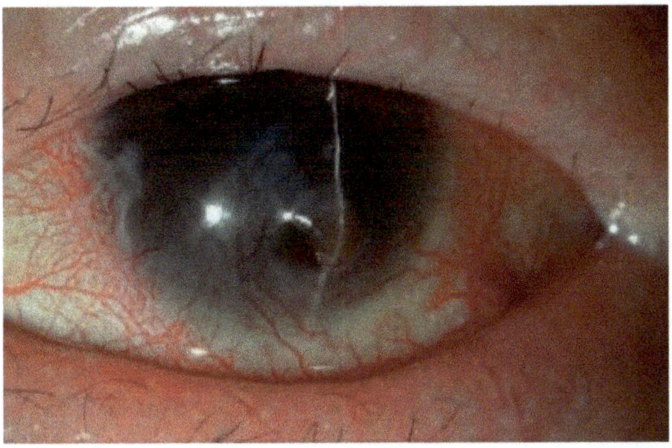

**Figure 136.** Severe ocular rosacea can sometimes lead to corneal perforation, which in turn leads to the release of aqueous humor.

absence of CD does not mean that the patient does not have ocular rosacea; sometimes imago-stage Demodex are eliminated, but their eggs remain at the eyelash root, causing the patient to experience recurring symptoms. Additionally, if a patient experiences recurrent symptoms of chalazia or if a severe chalazion causes the ectropion or deformity of the eyelid, it may indicate the presence of ocular rosacea.

**The clinical signs and symptoms of ocular rosacea may include the following in one or both eyes:**

Red eyes
Burning sensation
Itching and tearing
Dryness
Foreign body sensation
Blurred vision
Photosensitivity or photophobia
Conjunctival neovascularization or capillary dilation
Recurrent inflammation of the eyelid
Repeated infection of the ocular surface or eyelid, including conjunctivitis, blepharitis, and styes (hordeolum) or chalazion.

## 6.3 Diagnosis

### 6.3.1 *Differential diagnosis of ocular rosacea*

Ocular rosacea was officially declared as fourth subtype (or type IV) of rosacea by the NRS in 2002.[1] The 2017 global ROSCO panel states that phenotype is the metric by which the diagnosis, classification, and treatments for rosacea should be made. The panel categorized rosacea phenotype by diagnostic features, major feature and minor or secondary feature. The 2019 ROSCO panel further introduced supplementary descriptions of ocular rosacea characteristics to aid in the diagnosis and assessment.

Ocular rosacea has specific manifestations in the eye that act as diagnostic characteristics, and the major features are marginal vascular filaments of the eyelid, blepharitis, keratitis/conjunctivitis/sclerokeratitis (conjunctival hyperemia of the eyelids, spade-like infiltration of the cornea, scleritis, sclerokeratitis, and corneal neovascularization), and other ocular symptoms. The minor or secondary features are honey-like scale crust at the eyelash root, irregular eyelid edge, and rapid evaporation of tears.

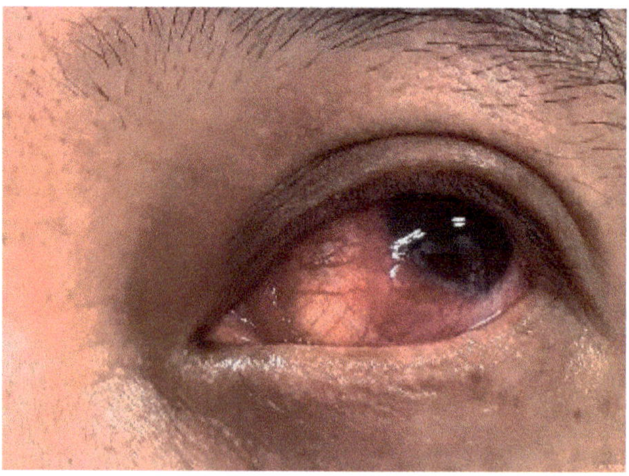

**Figure 137.** Scleritis caused by Demodex

### 6.3.2 *Treatment*

In terms of the treatment of ocular rosacea, in addition to the vital first step of determining whether the ocular rosacea is due to an ocular Demodex infestation, and if it is determined that the patient may have the said Demodex infestation, appropriate drugs will be administered to target the mites once further tests confirm the diagnosis. The eye is a highly sensitive area and cannot be treated using newly developed dermatological medications or ointments which would irritate the eye. The principle of treatment generally begins from conservative management, first focusing on understanding whether a patient has underlying DES, MGD, or any other similar eye disease. Treatment includes the application of hot compresses; use of artificial teardrops, gels, or ointments; and ensuring that patients avoid contact lenses for a prolonged duration. In terms of topical, localized, antimicrobial products, typical drugs include tetracycline ointment, erythromycin, or even metronidazole, azithromycin, bacitracin, polymyxin B, or fusidic acid. In terms of other types of medication, ibuprofen is commonly used as an anti-inflammatory agent, whereas steroids are only recommended during the acute stage of the condition. Prolonged use of steroids is recommended to prevent complications such as glaucoma or cataracts. Additionally, because the symptoms of ocular rosacea have a high degree of overlap with other ophthalmic conditions, medications targeted at other such conditions may be used in combination. These include topical cyclosporine, which is used for grade 2 or higher DES, which may also be useful in treating ocular rosacea. In terms of oral medications, despite there being a wide variety of drugs available to select from, the most commonly used and most effective drug, doxycycline, will generally suffice.

In terms of treatment, the clinical symptoms associated with Demodex infestations are reversible if treated as early as possible. In summary, although the triggers causing ocular rosacea are complex and similar to those which cause rosacea of the skin, a conclusion has not yet been reached as to whether ocular rosacea is entirely due to Demodex infestation, though there is certainly a close correlation. Clinical experience has shown that although some patients may have no visible signs of blepharitis or Demodex, clinical indications and microscopic testing of plucked eyelashes show Demodex deep within the hair follicle; thus, it would be incorrect to rule out Demodex. One of the most overlooked triggers causing such different manifestations of Demodex is that there is a strong correlation between the clinical manifestations and each individual's facial cleansing habits. In terms of the strategy for the treatment of Demodex infestations, the most important factor is to screen Demodex mites to identify patients with Demodex infestation, find a method to halt the vicious cycle, and improve the clinical symptoms for these patients. However, because Demodex can hide deep inside pores and eyelash follicles, medication is usually only able to eliminate Demodex closer to the surface. Relying solely upon medication for elimination will result in limited effectiveness; thus, we recommend combining the medication with cleansing and hot compresses to bring Demodex to the surface where they can be killed. Additionally, the treatment of Demodex infestations is also very helpful at treating ocular rosacea and controlling the condition. Although no complete cure currently exists for ocular rosacea, medication and adequate eye care can help control the appearance and symptoms of the condition.

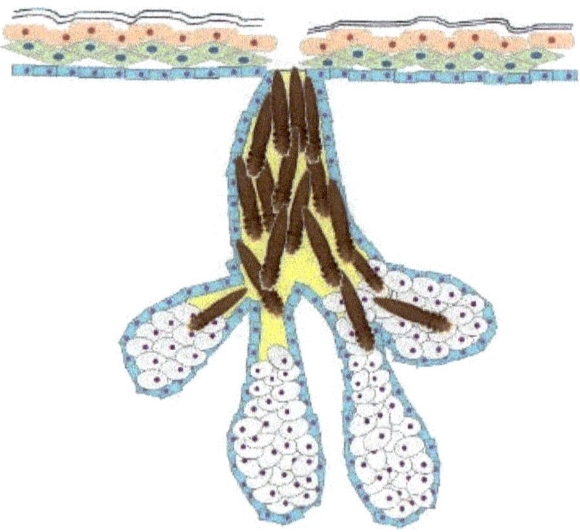

**Figure 138.** Demodex skin infestations may be just the tip of the iceberg, and there may be more to it than that meets the eye.

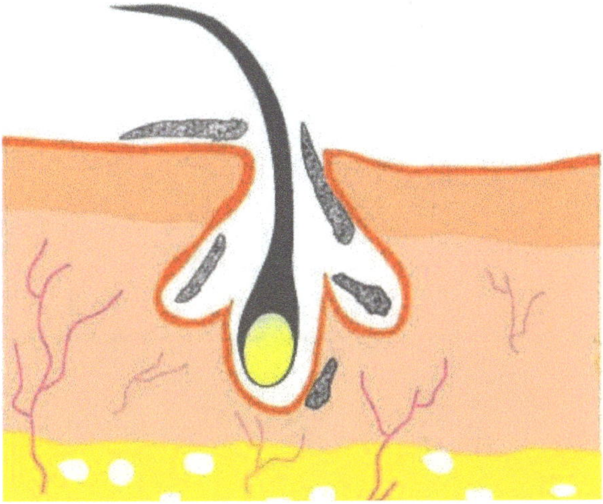

**Figure 139.** Demodex infestation at the base of the eyelash follicle may be more serious than meets the eye, just like the tip of the iceberg.

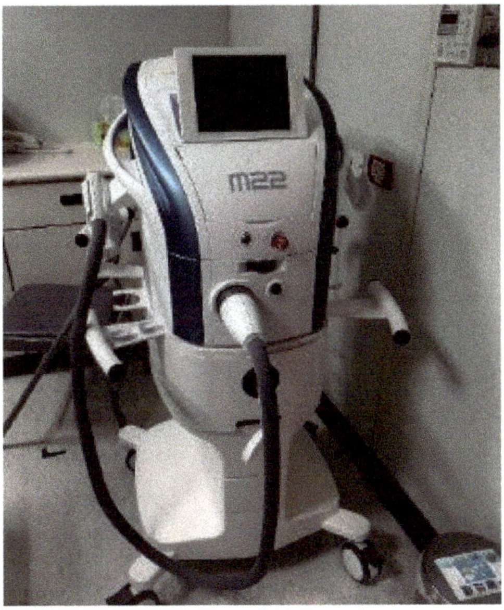


**Figure 140.** Lumenis® M22TM IPL system.

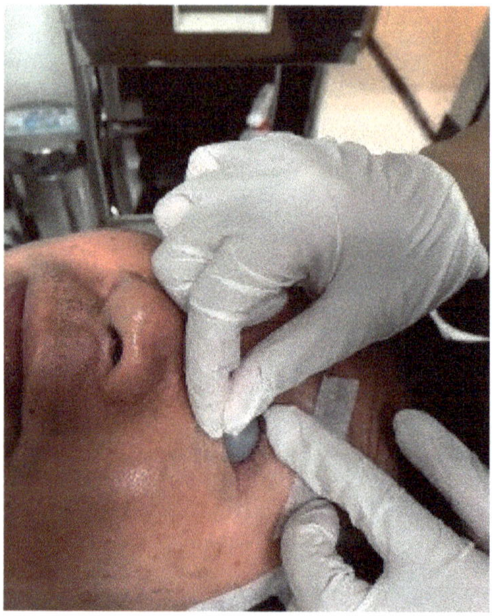

**Figure 141.** Protect the surface of the eye while using the Lumenis M22TM IPL system.

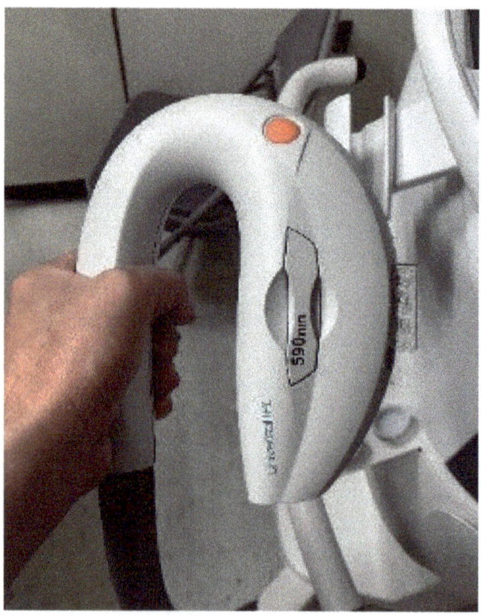


**Figure 142.** Select a filter using the Lumenis M22TM IPL system.

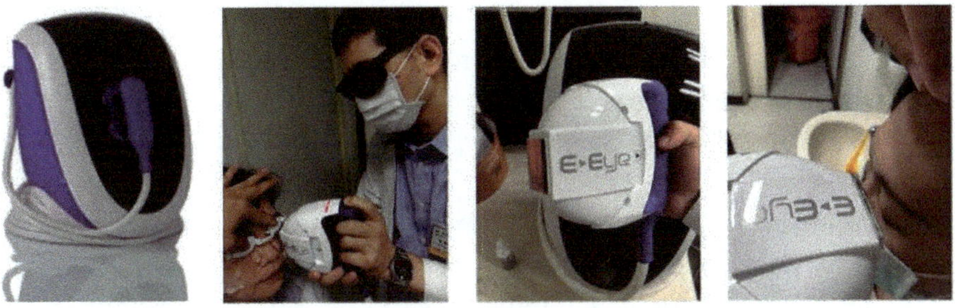

**Figure 143.** EYE IPL machine system.

Pulsed light laser treatment for rosacea of the skin: IPL lasers differ from single-wavelength lasers, as they produce a wave band of 400–1200 nm. The light ray within the wave band is used for selective photothermal decomposition, achieving blemish removal, vascular filament removal, hair removal, and skin rejuvenation.

Key points and information regarding postoperative care for pulsed light treatment:

1. For patients who are allergic to anesthesia, have a history of herpes simplex, have a heart condition, or who are pregnant, the doctor should be informed.
2. For patients who have used isotretinoin or photosensitizing medication in the 2 weeks prior to treatment or have been exposed to excessive sunlight in the past month, it is important to inform the doctor.
3. In the event of a bacterial or viral infection of the skin, inform the doctor.
4. The number of treatment courses required and their efficacy will depend upon skin color and treatment type. Spots, pigmentation, and vascular filaments may require multiple treatments to visibly improve and sometimes require combination with other treatments to achieve optimal results.
5. Skin reacts differently depending on the symptoms. Slightly red skin accompanied by a warm sensation may persist for 0.5–1 h.
6. By the following day, most spots will have formed into scabs and will fall off within a week. The scabs are allowed to fall naturally, and once they fall, the spots have been eliminated completely.

7. Telangiectasia: After treatment, blood vessels become darker, and slight redness and inflammation around the blood vessels are normal. The photothermal laser destroys the blood vessels which are then naturally metabolized by the body, becoming invisible after around a week.
8. Rosacea of the skin: After treatment, the skin will likely be more flushed than that prior to the treatment, but after a period of time, the redness will subside. If the redness is too visible, an ice pack can be used to bring the flushing down rapidly.
9. Makeup can be applied after treatment in the absence of post-treatment wounds and adverse skin reactions.
10. Moisturization and sunscreen are essential for post-treatment care.
11. Moisturization accelerates skin metabolic repair, whereas sunscreen protects the skin against secondary burning caused by UV radiation.
12. For 2 days after treatment, skincare products with irritating ingredients, such as alcohol and whitening products, should not be used. It is also important to avoid activities which may cause skin irritation, such as sunbathing, bathing in a hot spring or spa, or intense exercise.

## References

1. Rather PA, Hassan I. Human *Demodex* mite: the versatile mite of dermatological importance. *J Dermatol.* 2014;59(1):60–66.
2. Baudouin C, Messmer EM, Aragona P, et al. Revisiting the vicious circle of dry eye disease: a focus on the pathophysiology of meibomian gland dysfunction. *Br J Ophthalmol.* 2016;100:300–306.
3. Blackie CA, Solomon JD, Greiner JV, Holmes M, Korb DR. Inner eyelid surface temperature as a function of warm compress methodology. *Optom Vis Sci.* 2008;85(8):675–83.
4. Mori A, Shimazaki J, Shimmura S, Fujishima H, Oguchi Y, Tsubota K. Disposable eyelid-warming device for the treatment of meibomian gland dysfunction. *Jpn J Ophthalmol.* 2003;47:578–586.
5. Olson MC, Korb DR, Greiner JV. Increase in tear film lipid layer thickness following treatment with warm compresses in patients with meibomian gland dysfunction. *Eye Contact Lens.* 2003;29(2):96–9.
6. Goto E, Monden Y, Takano Y, Mori A, Shimmura S, Shimazaki J, Tsubota K. Treatment of non-inflamed obstructive meibomian gland

dysfunction by an infrared warm compression device. *Br J Ophthalmol.* 2002;86(12):1403–7.

7. Murphy O, O'Dwyer V, Lloyd-McKernan A. Ocular Demodex folliculorum: prevalence and associated symptoms in an Irish population. *Int Ophthalmol.* 2019;39(2):405–417.
8. Gao YY, Di Pascuale MA, Li W, Liu DT, Baradaran-Rafii A, Elizondo A, Kawakita T, Raju VK, Tseng SC. High prevalence of Demodex in eyelashes with cylindrical dandruff. *Invest Ophthalmol Vis Sci.* 2005;46:3089–94.
9. Liu J, Sheha H, Tseng SC. Pathogenic role of Demodex mites in blepharitis. *Curr Opin Allergy Clin Immunol.* 2010;10(5):505–10.
10. Czepita D, Kuźna-Grygiel W, Kosik-Bogacka D. Badania nad wystepowaniem oraz rola Demodex folliculorum i Demodex brevis w patogenezie przewlekłego zapalenia brzegów powiek [Investigations on the occurrence as well as the role of Demodex follicuforum and Demodex brevis in the pathogensis of blepharitis]. *Klin Oczna.* 2005;107(1–3):80–2.
11. Gao YY, Di Pascuale MA, Li W, Baradaran-Rafii A, Elizondo A, Kuo CL, Raju VK, Tseng SC. In vitro and in vivo killing of ocular Demodex by tea tree oil. *Br J Ophthalmol.* 2005;89(11):1468–1473.
12. Tighe S, Gao YY, Tseng SC. Terpinen-4-ol is the most active ingredient of tea tree oil to kill Demodex mites. *Transl Vis Sci Technol.* 2013;2(7):2.
13. Murphy O, O'Dwyer V, Lloyd-McKernan A. The efficacy of tea tree face wash, 1, 2-Octanediol and microblepharoexfoliation in treating *Demodex folliculorum* blepharitis. *Cont Lens Anterior Eye.* 2018;41(1):77–82.
14. Ngo W, Jones L, Bitton E. Short-term comfort responses associated with the use of eyelid cleansing products to manage *Demodex folliculorum. Eye Contact Lens.* 2018;44(Suppl 2):S87-S92.
15. Yun SH, Levin F, Servat J. Demodex folliculitis presenting as periocular vesiculopustular rash. *Orbit.* 2013;32(6):370–1.
16. Hung KH, Lan YH, Lin JY, Kang EY, Tan HY, Chen HC, Hsiao CH, Yeh LK. Potential role and significance of ocular demodicosis in patients with concomitant refractory herpetic keratitis. *Clin Ophthalmol.* 2020;14:4469–4482.
17. Hung KH, Tan HY, Chen HC, Yeh LK. Clinical characteristics and topographic findings of corneal ectasia in patients with symptomatic *Demodex* blepharitis. *Taiwan J Ophthalmol.* 2020;11(2):146–155.
18. Zhao YE, Guo N, Wu LP. The effect of temperature on the viability of *Demodex folliculorum* and *Demodex brevis. Parasitol Res.* 2009;105: 1623–1628.

# Special Thanks

⑩ Emotional stories from patients with rosacea

One

When I stepped into Dr. Huang's clinic one February morning in 2014, the clinic was full of other patients waiting to be seen. Even the nurses at the entrance desk seemed incredibly busy.

When it was my turn to see the doctor, I sat down in the consulting chair and suddenly went from holding back tears to beginning to cry hysterically. I said to Dr. Huang, "The medicine you prescribed me smells so bad, and it really hurts. This week I have been so worried that someone would smell the medicine on me and might think that I stink and I am unhygienic. I am a music teacher, so my students are often in close contact with me. I am afraid that my students will think that their teacher smells strange." I hated this so much, because I am so obsessed with cleanliness!

I did not care that I was surrounded by nurses. I just could not stop crying. Dr. Huang sat down opposite me and after listening to me complain and vent with so much patience and compassion, he responded in a warm tone, "It is okay, teacher X. We will think of another solution."

Upon hearing Dr. Huang's words, I felt as if I had been rescued, and I slowly began to calm down. After wiping away my tears, I thanked Dr. Huang and began to slowly open the door and walk out of the examination room. Ah! In an instant, dozens of pairs of curious eyes fixated their attention onto me. Before it was my turn to see the doctor, every seat in the clinic had been taken, but now even the narrow corridor was crowded with patients. As I left the examination room, I brushed past the crowds of people and wanted to avoid their gazes, lowering my head to instead search for my phone in my bag. It was only when I turned on my phone that I realized that half an hour had passed since I went in to see the doctor!

That morning was certainly unforgettable for me.

"We have finally figured out a way to eliminate the pain, when you use Jaline lotion, and the smell of the anti-Demodex treatment," Dr. Huang told me in a cheerful yet determined tone. "The Jaline lotion and the tea tree oil should be applied in sequence. The pain completely disappears, and the smell will be covered. The essential oil does not have a bad smell and does have a certain effect. Then, we combine this with a laser treatment to target erythema and blood vessels." Later, I learned that in the previous 4 days, Dr. Huang had tried using many maintenance products with Jaline lotion, but none had achieved the desired effects. The treatment was not successful until he finally tried using tea tree oil. I really admire Dr. Huang's dedication and efficiency.

My experience of treatment was as follows: In January 2014, I discovered that I had rosacea with Demodex. In February, I was prescribed Jaline lotion for treatment, but within a week I could not stand the pain and smell of the medication. Four days later, I was prescribed Jaline lotion combined with tea tree oil and a supplementary treatment of a pulsed dye laser and dual wavelength laser. Four months later, my face appeared much brighter, and no Demodex could be detected.

In 2018, my Demodex problem recurred, so I began to use ivermectin cream as treatment. In 2021, I began using a repair essence for those with rosacea-prone skin, and in 2022, I started Sylfirm treatment. Prior to my Sylfirm treatment, I was assessed for Demodex once more, which confirmed that no Demodex could be found on my skin!

I have no itching or flushing issues on my skin anymore. Additionally, using Sylfirm to stabilize and repair my skin after treatment is the best experience I have ever felt.

However, throughout the treatment process, the unknown has led to me experiencing a lot of fear about what may happen. But now, after experiencing the treatment process, I know that it has been successful and that there is an end point. My skin today has not been negatively affected by the treatment of Demodex. Because I am continuing to maintain and care for my skin, it has remained in a condition that I am very happy with!

Of course, if I ever encounter any other skin issues, I would have complete trust in Dr. Huang's treatments and advice.

Two

The first time I attended Dr. Huang's clinic was in 2013, when I was diagnosed with rosacea and an excess of Demodex mites, and I was prescribed an anti-Demodex medication as treatment. However, after a week of treatment, I felt like my rosacea had not improved at all. I stopped going to the clinic and just decided I would have to live with the remaining rosacea.

After I retired in June 2022, I increased the frequency and intensity of my exercise; consequently, my rosacea worsened. My facial skin was red and hot after I exercised and would take a long time to return to normal. I decided to return to Dr. Huang's clinic and received the same diagnosis as I had obtained in 2013, an excess of Demodex and rosacea. This time, I followed Dr. Huang's advice and used the Soolantra cream paired with a skincare serum developed by Dr. Huang. With this treatment, I found that the redness and heat of my face after exercise had been alleviated, and I did not get rosacea flare-ups after exercise anymore. My skin was able to remain stable after exercise. I am so happy that I do not have to make a choice between my physical health and my skin anymore. In addition, Dr. Huang also discovered during treatment that the hypertension medication that I take daily causes vasodilation, which worsens my rosacea. Subsequently, I visited my family physician to get my medication changed to the one which would not have the same side effects.

After following Dr. Huang's treatment plan for the past few months, I definitely feel that he is an incredibly patient and a skilled doctor. Through our daily consultation, I was able to discover that my hypertension medication could have been exacerbating my rosacea. When I felt a prickling sensation in my nose, Dr. Huang was able to explain the mechanism causing this sensation and helped me treat it and eliminate such a painful symptom of my condition. Dr. Huang always says, "Medicine must be precise." Therefore, Dr. Huang is very careful and attentive in his actions including sampling, research, or treatment, and he has extensive background knowledge of the relevant issues. I am incredibly lucky to be able to work with Dr. Huang to take care of my skin and solve the rosacea issue that has been bothering me for >10 years.

I really admire the depth and breadth of his medical knowledge. I also wish to recommend Dr. Huang to everybody so that more people will get to understand his medical skills. I would also love for him to become famous in Tainan, or even Taiwan as a whole so that people from Taiwan and abroad with dermatological concerns will hear about him and be able to visit the clinic for treatment.

Three

Congratulations to Dr. Huang on publishing his book. As for sharing my story, there really is nothing much to share, as I am mostly just fed up with Demodex!

I have repeated breakouts of Demodex with no clear cause, and there is no permanent cure for the time being. Because constitution differs between individuals, there are no preventive measures that can be taken, so I just have to get treated passively whenever I have an outbreak. This is really disruptive to my life.

I feel like Demodex is similar to herpes simplex; once you have had one outbreak, you will have to deal with it for the rest of your life. However, Demodex is even more problematic than herpes in some ways because herpes at least stops fighting back against the host, whereas Demodex does not. They just keep attacking, causing the skin to keep reacting in some way.

Usually, when the outbreak is not serious, it causes facial flushing or local erythema, but this can also grow into small pustules, usually as few as two or three; however, in more serious cases there can be up to ten pustules scattered across the face.

For example, I repeatedly develop small pustules and flushing on my nose, with the most worrisome being those that develop on my eyelids, because they take the longest time and are the most painful to allow to heal naturally without follow-up treatment.

I mostly worry about hot weather. In the hot weather, a slight redness spreads out across my face, or I might get localized allergic reactions. In severe cases, I feel a noticeable burning and constant irritating sensations as if I am being pricked by needles.

Finally, the most common, yet relatively minor symptom is of itching. My face constantly feels itchy, with no particular time, season, or weather that seems to cause it.

Thus, on the whole, I feel irritable, bored with this condition, and inconvenienced. I feel so discouraged when I experience a flare-up, and while my mood is never completely negative, I still feel quite depressed.

That is my experience with this condition.

A note from Dr. Huang: Prior to attending our clinic, this patient was misdiagnosed and prescribed a steroid cream treatment for several months. After only one day of not using this medication, the patient experienced a breakout of papulopustules. After 4 months of treatment in our clinic, we were able to restore brightness to the skin and reduce redness of the skin until it was only faint. For over a year afterwards, the patient experienced repeated idiopathic superficial folliculitis of the face and did not return to our clinic for 7 months. At the time at which we invited the patient to share their story, we invited them back to the clinic for assessment. We discovered an excess of Demodex and provided further treatment, and after 3 months the patient's condition had stabilized.

www.ingramcontent.com/pod-product-compliance
Lightning Source LLC
LaVergne TN
LVHW051056210926
848486LV00002B/121
* 9 7 8 9 8 1 9 8 2 7 8 8 6 *